THE IRON DISORDERS INSTITUTE
Guide to
HEMOCHROMATOSIS

THE IRON DISORDERS INSTITUTE
Guide to
HEMOCHROMATOSIS

Edited by Cheryl D. Garrison,
Iron Disorders Institute Cofounder

Scientific Advisors
Wylie Burke, PH.D., M.D.; P. D. Phatak, M.D.;
E. D. Weinberg, PH.D.

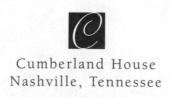

Cumberland House
Nashville, Tennessee

Published by Cumberland House Publishing, Inc., 431 Harding Industrial Drive, Nashville, TN 37211

Cover design: Gore Studios, Inc.

Advisors and contributing scientists are not responsible for the contents of *Guide to Hemochromatosis*. This book is an Iron Disorders Institute publication and not the sole work of any advisor, contributing scientist, or other person. Contents of *The Iron Disorders Institute Guide to Hemochromatosis* are for informational purposes and not intended to replace the advice of one's physician.

Library of Congress Cataloging-in-Publication Data

The Iron Disorders Institute guide to hemochromatosis / Cheryl Garrison, editor.
    p. cm.
"Scientific advisors, Wylie Burke, P. D. Phatak, E. D. Weinberg."
Includes bibliographical references and index.
ISBN 1-58182-160-3 (alk. paper)
    1. Hemochromatosis--Popular works. I. Garrison, Cheryl, 1945–
II. Iron Disorders Institute.

RC632.H4 I76 2001
616.3'96--dc21

2001028136

Printed in the United States of America
1 2 3 4 5 6 7—05 04 03 02 01 00

Dedication

To Webb B. Garrison Sr. (July 1919–July 2000), a world-renowned writer of Civil War books. Mr. Garrison did not have hemochromatosis, but his wisdom, thoughtfulness, and encouragement made a book about this disorder possible.

Contents

Foreword

Until the discovery of HFE gene and its mutations, hereditary hemochromatosis (HH) was not a commonly diagnosed condition. However, we now know that HH is the leading cause of iron overload disease and the most common hereditary disease that affects Caucasians of Northern European ancestry. The common form of HH is due to a mutation at a single point in a gene that has been called the HFE gene. Two of these mutations must usually be present in a person (an autosomal recessive condition) in order for the person to develop heavy iron overload. Such persons have life-long excessive intestinal absorption of iron, which leads to deposition of the metal in the liver, heart, pancreas, and other organs. Excess iron may be toxic and even fatal. Timely diagnosis of hereditary hemochromatosis and treatment with phlebotomy can prevent this organ damage. Physicians can perform a simple blood test to determine if a patient is at risk for iron overload. This test is the serum transferrin iron saturation percentage (TS%). If TS% is elevated above 55%, the test should be repeated fasting. If the fasting TS% is greater than 45%, the physician and patient should suspect iron overload and proceed with additional tests such as serum ferritin and HFE gene mutational analysis.

Two mutations in the HFE gene have been linked to the hemochromatosis phenotype; the major mutation is called C282Y and the minor mutation (less strongly associated with HH and with milder forms of HH), called H63D. Iron overload occurs chiefly in persons who are homozygous for the C282Y mutation (C282Y +/+) and, less often in those who are heterozygous for both C282Y and H63D (C282Y +/- AND H63D -/+). Tests for both are now widely and commercially available, and these tests have helped to establish definitive diagnoses, particularly in patients and their families with the classic form of hereditary hemochromatosis.

In the United States about 80–85 percent of patients with iron overload have the mutations in the HFE gene associated with HH. In addition, some persons who are homozygous abnormal for the major mutation (C282Y +/+), especially women, do not express the iron overload phenotype. Then, too, there are clearly other types of hereditary hemochromatosis (e.g., those occurring in black Africans or Melanesians), in which causative mutations occur in other, still unidentified genes.

Prior to discovery of the HFE gene and identification of the major mutations that cause HH, physicians relied on liver biopsy for diagnosis because the liver is the principal organ responsible for the storage and detoxification of iron. It is also the first and foremost organ damaged by heavy iron overload. Indeed, the "gold standard" for the diagnosis of iron overload is still liver biopsy with determination of the hepatic iron index. This index is defined as the hepatic iron concentration, expressed as micromoles of iron per gram of dry liver, divided by the age of the patient in years. Values greater than 1.9 are indicative of HH. Liver biopsy, however, is invasive and rarely may be associated with complications. Furthermore, the variability in measured hepatic iron concentrations in small liver samples from patients with cirrhosis may be considerable. Genetic testing has revolutionized diagnosis of HH because we can now make firm diagnoses in most patients without liver biopsies. Biopsies continue to be important to assess the presence and severity of hepatic fibrosis (scar tissue), but, among C282Y +/+ patients, without elevated liver enzymes in the serum (AST, ALT), without abnormal livers on physical examination, and with serum ferritin levels less than 1000 ng/mL, we now know that such patients will never have cirrhosis or advanced fibrosis on biopsy. We also have made progress in developing non-invasive methods for estimating the hepatic iron concentrations. A dedicated device to measure magnetic susceptibilities, the superconducting quantum interference device, is accurate for the estimation of hepatic iron concentrations but is not widely available. Although computed tomography (CT scanning) demonstrates an increase in the attenuation of the liver in hepatic iron overload, it is relatively insensitive to mild degrees of increased hepatic iron, especially if there is associated fatty change in the liver. Special magnetic resonance (MR) imaging is a more promising noninvasive modality to estimate hepatic iron concentration. An increase in hepatic iron concentration decreases the T2 relaxation time, which decreases the liver's signal intensity and makes the liver appear dark on typical MR images.

Diagnostic breakthrough approaches such as HFE DNA analysis and specialized MRI are revolutionizing the way we can help persons with conditions of excessive tissue iron. We are still on the threshold of understanding the many details and intricacies of iron metabolism. We need additional studies of the duodenum (the main site of iron absorption), liver, pancreas, heart, joints, and brain (especially the pituitary gland) and how iron-mediated damage contributes to chronic diseases such as atherosclerosis, cancer, chronic viral hepatitis, and other liver diseases. More studies on diet are needed to help us better understand the bioavailability and absorption of iron and which dietary measures to decrease iron absorption work and which do not.

Joint efforts by the scientific community, the medical community, governmental health resources (CDC, NIH and others), private industry, and national voluntary health agencies, such as the Iron Disorders Institute, can improve patient and physician education and research funding for such studies. Additional research and its translation into clinical care are the cornerstones for building further progress.

This book is designed particularly for patients with iron overload and their families. It provides up-to-date practical information, developed with laypersons in mind. The people at IDI, Cheryl Garrison, Chris Kieffer, and the president of IDI, Randy Alexander, deserve our thanks for the many hours of work that contributed to bringing this book to fruition.

—Herbert Bonkovsky, M.D., Director, Liver Center and Center for Study of Disorders of Iron and Porphyrin Metabolism, University of Massachusetts Medical School, Chairman, Iron Disorders Institute Scientific Advisory Board

Acknowledgments

Few people read long lists of acknowledgments; a reader's interest is directed at the main content of the book, as it should be. *The Iron Disorders Institute (IDI) Guide to Hemochromatosis* would not exist, however, without the names mentioned on this page of thanks.

As I think back over the last three years to events that contributed to this book, my first thoughts are of two very dear and generous men, Webb Garrison Sr., my father-in-law, and Eugene Weinberg, Professor of Microbiology, Indiana University and Scientific Advisory Board Chair, Publications. Without their patience, kindness, and generosity of time, this book would not exist.

My next thoughts are of two other special men, my husband, also named Webb Garrison, and my son, David. Webb never complained about my fourteen- or fifteen-hour days fixed at my computer. He tolerated faxes all hours of the day and weekend, as well as my time glued to the telephone, even while dinner he prepared grew cold and inedible. He took time from his own work to scan images, help me correct graphics, and finally to read the last version of the book and offer his opinion. If not for my son, David, I wouldn't be a cofounder of the Iron Disorders Institute, and I would not know many of the fine people mentioned in this acknowledgment page, or within the pages of this book. David has an iron loading condition, and through his experience, I have learned.

Chris Kieffer comes to mind next. "Cheryl, our work will have an effect on world health! Think of the people we can help!" Chris would always interject into our conversations. For her hours on the phone chasing down facts and details, including securing the first public comment from the U.S. Surgeon General about iron overload, I thank you, Chris. Next, I'd like to thank Randy Alexander; for without his experience with hemochromatosis, and his ability to persevere in the face of personal sacrifices and undeserved ridicule, attention to this health issue would not exist at the levels it does today.

Besides helping immeasurably with sections of the book by editing, copywriting, and designing graphics or by offering inspiration and support, the next people I mention added the final touches that brought the entire project together. These people are Ron Pitkin, Bruce Gore, who designed a spectacular jacket cover, and Lisa Taylor for her editing talents, all of Cumberland House Publishing. Fran Weinberg, Kay and Mickey Owen, Donna Duncan, Dolores and Bob Forman, Laura, Dick and Matthew Main, Missy Kendall, Mary Jane Thomson, Bonnie Ritter, Sandy and Jeff Bowers, Julie Stegall, Ron DeKett, Ellie Leuthie, Jen Opperman, John McGruder, Barbara Taylor, Cliff Stitcher, Dr. Shel Reyes, Dr. William Dietz, Dr. Stephen Nightingale, Dr. David Sundwall, the entire IDI Scientific Advisory Board, especially Dr. Herbert Bonkovsky, and Dr. Prad Phatak, Dr. Vincent Felitti, Naomi Howard, Dr. Sharon McDonnell, Dr. Elizabeth Thomson and her great assistant Sue, Dr. Priscilla Short, Dr. Phyllis Sholinsky, Dr. H. Ralph Schumacher, Dr. Joe McCord, Dr. Barbara Bowman, Dr. Louis Heck, Dr. Daniel Bailey, and companies that provided photographs of therapeutic equipment, Becton Dickinson, Sims Deltec-Medical Systems, and Baxter Healthcare.

When we put the call out for personal stories, they poured into our headquarters by the hundreds. We read each and every story; all of them are compelling, some heartwarming, some sad, some are funny and uplifting. I wish we could have used all of them, but I especially want to thank: Rosalie Yee, Bobby Montgomery, Johnny Taylor, Tom Mowell, Betty Thomas, David Remer, David Kitzman, and Larry Archibald. Chris and I enjoyed the interviews we had with you. Ruth Oakes and her husband's story is one I especially cherish. These stories will not go untold; they will be published in the very near future in our magazine or in another book.

Regards,
Cheryl Garrison, Cofounder, Iron Disorders Institute,
Vice President, Educational Product Development

Introduction: A Message from the Founders of the Iron Disorders Institute

The Iron Disorders Institute was originally called the Common Ground Institute. It was so named because we as founders knew that all entities related to the health issue of hemochromatosis would have to work together to address problems such as medical community and public awareness, consensus on issues where discrepancies remained, and to produce quality educational materials. Many told us we were crazy if we thought we could get people to work together toward a common set of goals; it would be impossible. We disagreed and pressed on, contacting some of the most inaccessible people in the country (and the world) for their perspectives. When our book became a reality, we had solid proof that getting people to work together toward a common set of goals is not an impossible dream. This book contains the best of hundreds of thousands of words and numerous meaningful images as a result of this cooperative spirit.

As you read *The Iron Disorders Institute Guide to Hemochromatosis*, we want you to know how much heart, caring, and personal sacrifice helped to inspire and shape its contents. In this message from us, the founders of the Iron Disorders Institute, we share what motivated us to dedicate ourselves to helping others with projects such as this book.

Randy S. Alexander, Founder, Iron Disorders Institute
"I have hemochromatosis. I know firsthand what many of you who also have this condition have endured. For years now, the majority of us with hemochromatosis have had to live with pain,

hardship, loss, sadness, and frustration because of the incorrect notion that the disorder is obscure and rare. When I was trying to get diagnosed, information was scarce and much of its content questionable. There seemed to be few real medical experts addressing this health issue.

"Hemochromatosis claimed the life of my father with a heart attack at age fifty-nine; it then began to claim my health, and the health of one of my brothers and my only sister. My mother suffered because of the struggles of ill health, and the emotional devastation of seeing her family wither away right before her eyes. At times it was unbearable for her. The search for answers and the task of trying to inform others was, at times, simply maddening. As an advocate, perseverance was all that I had to keep me going.

"My message about this disorder was clear: 'It's real, it's common, and it can kill you' if not properly diagnosed and treated. Because hemochromatosis is treatable, early intervention can result in the prevention of chronic disease. This alone makes hemochromatosis, without question, a powerful model for preventive health care."

Chris L. Kieffer, Cofounder, Iron Disorders Institute
"My husband, Harry, has hemochromatosis. Trying to get him diagnosed and the best treatment was very frustrating. We were shocked that the medical community did not have the latest information on iron overload.

"The most common genetic disorder was being almost totally overlooked and misunderstood, and I was appalled. Harry could have eventually died if I hadn't kept pushing and asking questions and digging for answers: That is my style—get motivated to get things done. The direction of our lives has changed forever. We now have a mission in life to help others with what we have endured. That is why we founded IDI. Our efforts have not gone unrewarded; when people tell us how much we have helped them, we know that all the sacrifices are worth it and that we are on the right track. What else in life could we do that would be that rewarding? What we are working on can have a major affect on world health and disease prevention; of this I am certain. My hope is that this book will help you and your family to understand iron overload and save you valuable time spent researching and in frustration, and enable you to be proactive and work with your physician. My husband had a positive out-come; others can too. It's so common that we all know someone with iron overload. *Don't* keep this information a secret; you, too, could help save lives!"

Cheryl D. Garrison, Cofounder, Iron Disorders Institute
"My son David was diagnosed with hemochromatosis. He exem-plifies the complexities of an iron overload condition because he doesn't fit the typical profile of hereditary hemochromatosis. He loads iron rapidly, and did so at a much younger age than most. He was fifteen when I first heard the word *hemochromatosis*. I have learned so much through him, and with this I feel I have been able to help other mothers who worry about their children. I swallow hard when I tell them not to worry, because I remem-ber how it felt to deal with the unknowns. My son was very ill, and I thought the worst—that he was going to die before doc-tors could figure out what was wrong with him. There is so much we have yet to learn about hemochromatosis and other iron loading disorders. What I do know for sure is that questions about this condition cannot be addressed with simple answers."

Hemochromatosis is not a new word, but when asked to define this condition, we find ourselves charged with a complicated task. Do we define it by symptoms? We cannot. We know certain symptoms accompany this condition, but symptoms manifest differently in people. So, do we define the condition with blood test results? People with hemochromatosis display differences here too. Some are actually anemic but have excess tissue iron. The gene for hemochromatosis was discovered in 1996. What if we use the genetic makeup to define hemochromatosis? This method, too, has limitations.

As we shaped *The Iron Disorders Institute Guide to Hemochro-matosis*, we turned to people who are living with the disorder for guidance. We read and reread hundreds of fine scientific papers. We talked with scientists all over the world. We listened, and then we took all these perspectives into consideration combined with our own experiences with hemochromatosis. This led us to the conclusion that hemochromatosis would be better under-stood within the matrix of iron disorders.

Many scientists are familiar with the term "hemochromato-sis"; yet, much of the medical profession is just beginning to learn the meaning of the word. Centuries of being focused on iron deficiencies have created a "one-sided" view of iron. Emerging technologies, and educational programs and materials are adding new dimensions to long-established belief systems regarding this important metal. Decades of ignorance about the extent to which excess iron can destroy health and unnecessarily claim the lives of husbands, wives, children, parents, and siblings are, we trust, coming to an end.

Modern medicine is armed with technology that now can identify the gene mutations for this disorder. U.S. Surgeon General Dr. David Satcher has acknowledged that hemochromatosis/iron overload provides an excellent opportunity for prevention of chronic disease. Our government health agencies have begun distribution of educational materials to the medical community and have provided funding for research to study hemochromatosis/iron overload. There is a simple blood test that can be used to detect excessive levels of tissue iron. Therapy is affordable, and now patients have a current and comprehensive handbook, *The Iron Disorders Institute Guide to Hemochromatosis*.

Patients have been able to obtain information through the Iron Disorders Institute's magazine, *idInsight*, and its praiseworthy website, www.irondisorders.org, for nearly four years. Now, IDI adds the first book, *The Iron Disorders Institute Guide to Hemochromatosis,* that can be used as a comprehensive home reference tool. Persons just diagnosed with hemochromatosis/iron overload will find the book a valuable resource for sensible diet planning, individualizing therapy, and learning the best way to detect iron problems in their children. Those who have had a long-term experience with hemochromatosis will enjoy reading compelling personal stories similar to their own. *The Guide to Hemochromatosis* can be used to help educate family members and physicians who remain skeptical about hemochromatosis. It includes helpful charts, treatment guidelines, diet suggestions, and a glossary of terms. This guide can empower patients to take charge of their health and work effectively with their physicians.

Throughout the *Guide to Hemochromatosis*, the reader will see italicized statements or bullet points. These points are intended to emphasize an issue or provide clarification of a possible lingering uncertainty. Referenced prominent surveys and special events appearing in shaded boxes include summary findings of the U.S. Centers for Disease Control and Prevention—1996 HHC Patient Survey, the European Association for the Study of the Liver (EASL) Consensus Conference on Hemochromatosis, and IRON2000 USA Scientific or Patient Conferences. These points appear in conjunction with personal stories that exemplify some of the problems experienced by people with iron imbalances such as hemochromatosis.

—Founders, Iron Disorders Institute:
Randy S. Alexander, Chris L. Kieffer,
and Cheryl D. Garrison

THE IRON DISORDERS INSTITUTE
Guide to
HEMOCHROMATOSIS

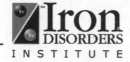
INSTITUTE

PART ONE

Iron—A Little Bit Goes a Long Way

"HEMOCHROMATOSIS, A DISORDER OF IRON METABOLISM, HAS BEEN DESCRIBED AS ONE OF MODERN MEDICINE'S BIGGEST OVERSIGHTS. . . ."

— *Dr. Randy Lauffer, author of* Iron and Your Heart, *St. Martin's Press, NYC*

Hemochromatosis: Not Just a Rare, Older Man's Disease

By the time John was thirty, he was impotent, depressed, exhausted, and experiencing severe chest pain. Before his fortieth birthday, he developed excruciating upper-right-quadrant abdominal pain, which added to his list of symptoms, now constant companions for John. He had seen five different private practice physicians, and been to the emergency room on twenty different occasions. Out of the countless number of doctors John encountered, most reached the same conclusion: he was a hypochondriac and needed psychiatric help. One physician, however, noted mildly elevated liver enzymes, and placed the note "hemochromatosis?" on John's chart but never mentioned the word or the test results. At age forty, John found himself undergoing shock treatment for severe depression. Addicted to Xanax™ and inconsolably sad, he added coppery-red-colored skin and severe heart palpitations to his expanding list of symptoms. John would not learn that he had hemochromatosis for another two years, at which time he would have advanced liver disease, permanent chronic fatigue, weakness, and extreme sensitivity to cold.

Once diagnosed, he thought back to his years in high school and recognized that delayed maturation and chest pain during his early twenties were part of the disease pattern for him. John is one of the numerous victims of undetected hemochromatosis. His disability and disease are due to years of unchecked iron accumulation, which was totally and absolutely preventable, if only his physician had been knowledgeable about iron and the disorder called hemochromatosis.

What Is Hemochromatosis?
Hemochromatosis is an inherited disorder of iron metabolism, not a blood disease. One might see the word spelled hemochromatosis, used by most people in the USA, or haemochromatosis, used widely abroad. Abbreviations for hemochromatosis include HH for hereditary hemochromatosis, HC for Hemochromatosis, GH for genetic hemochromatosis, and HHC for hereditary human hemochromatosis. Individuals who have this metabolic disorder do not regulate iron absorption normally. They can absorb as much as four times more iron from their diets than people with normal iron metabolism. Moreover, this iron cannot be excreted; therefore, over a period of three to five decades, iron accumulates to toxic levels in vital organs such as the liver, heart, joints, pancreas, brain, and pituitary gland.

This excessive iron burden leads to impaired function of these organs and eventually to disease and organ failure. Undetected and untreated, hemochromatosis can even be fatal.

Scientists know the liver is capable of accumulating large quantities of excess iron. It is often the first organ to fail in people with advanced hemochromatosis. How iron is distributed and accumulates within other body systems is not fully understood. Some of these other, smaller organs, such as the heart or the pituitary, may become damaged by smaller amounts of iron, resulting in weakness, heart arrhythmia, and hormonal imbalances before symptoms associated with liver disease occur. At the time these seemingly unrelated symptoms appear, the liver might actually be cirrhotic, while the patient can actually have no obvious signs of liver disease. John's story exemplifies this, as his first symptoms were hormonal and cardiac. Pain associated with liver disease did not manifest in John for seventeen years after his initial symptoms became noticeable. Typical hemochromatosis-related symptoms of joint pain and diabetes did not occur for John, even though he carries two copies of the most common mutation causing hemochromatosis, the C282Y mutation of the HFE gene.

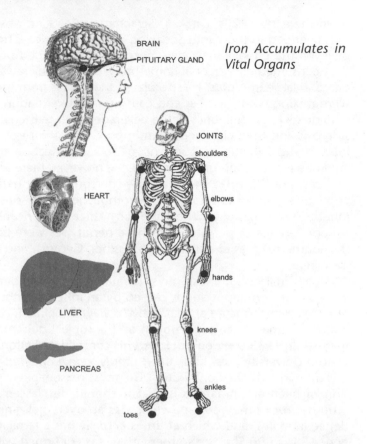

BRAIN
PITUITARY GLAND

Iron Accumulates in Vital Organs

JOINTS
shoulders

HEART

elbows

hands

LIVER

knees

PANCREAS

ankles

toes

Recognition of hemochromatosis can be traced back to the late nineteenth century. In 1889 a German scientist named H. von Recklinghausen noted a relationship between tissue injury, as in cirrhosis, and increased tissue iron. He termed this phenomenon "haemochromatosis," pronounced "hee-mo-chrom- oh-toe-sis"; *haem* for blood, *chroma* for bronze-colored skin, and *osis* for condition. A few years earlier in France, Dr. Armand Trousseau noted a relationship between skin color and diabetes. Due to the bronze coloring of skin, which seemed to accompany many of his diabetic patients, he named this condition "bronze diabetes." The terms "hemochromatosis" and "bronze diabetes" are still used interchangeably by many older clinicians and scientists.

In the early 1920s, Dr. A. S. Strachan of Scotland observed iron overload in the Bantu-speaking people of Africa. Strachan believed these individuals were becoming iron-loaded because they consumed a traditional home-brewed beer, which was prepared in large iron pots. He speculated that filings from the pots were mixing with the beer and causing iron overload in those who drank large quantities of the beverage. Later termed African siderosis and then classified as an important type of iron overload in sub-Saharan Africans, no genetic connection to HFE could be made in this group. In the USA, however, there are several cases of both HFE heterozygote (persons who inherit one copy of a gene mutation), and homozygote (persons who inherit two copies of a gene mutation) African Americans. The preponderance of persons with these genotypes were born in the southern states of Alabama, Mississippi, Georgia, and South Carolina.

Finally in 1927, a British physician named J. H. Sheldon suggested that iron deposition is caused by an inherited metabolic disorder. He conducted an exhaustive review of opinion, compiling all information he could obtain on the subject of hemochromatosis. In 1935 Sheldon published his consolidated effort in an Oxford University Press book titled simply, *Haemochromatosis*. In this monograph Sheldon wrote, "The most reasonable explanation of haemochromatosis is that it should be classed as an inborn error of metabolism, which has an overwhelming incidence in males, and which at times actually has a familial incidence." In 1996 Sheldon's observation was confirmed with the discovery of HFE, a principal gene for hereditary human hemochromatosis (HHC).

Discovery of HFE—The Gene for Hemochromatosis
While scientists searched for the hemochromatosis gene, centers worldwide were conducting hemochromatosis prevalence studies mostly using HLA typing—a method used to determine tissue compatibility by testing the saturation of iron-binding proteins in blood—or by liver biopsy. The *New England Journal of Medicine* published one of the first hemochromatosis incidence studies in 1988, "Prevalence of Hemochromatosis Among 11,065 Presumably Healthy Blood Donors," by noted clinicians and scientists

Edwards, Griffen, Goldgar, Drummond, Skolnick, and Kushner.

Results of this study, combined with results from similar incidence studies conducted in Australia, Finland, France, Germany, Spain, and Italy, substantiated the prevalence of hemochromatosis among those of Northern European descent to be 1 in about every 250 people. Those of Irish descent were found to have a prevalence of 1 in about 80. Still, much of the medical community remained unimpressed, until 1996 when a team of scientists at Mercator Genetics in California discovered HFE and two of its first known mutations, C282Y and H63D.

> "THE SCIENTIFIC COMMUNITY HAS SEARCHED FOR THIS GENE FOR TWENTY YEARS. . . ."
>
> —*Elliott Sigal, M.D., Ph.D., former CEO Mercator Genetics*

The gene discovery team of Feder, Gnirke, Thomas, Tsuchihashi, Ruddy, Basava, Dormishian, Domingo, Ellis, Fullan, Hinton, Jones, Kimmel, Kronmal, Lauer, Lee, Loeb, Mapa, McClelland, Meyer, Mintier, Moeller, Moore, Morikang, Prass, Quintana, Starnes, Schatzman, Brunke, Drayana, Rish, Bacon, and Wolff published their findings in *Nature Genetics* 1996. This breakthrough validated for people with hemochromatosis something they already knew to be true: Hemochromatosis is real, it's common, and it can be fatal.

Armed with modern technology, genetic analysis studies could now prove the frequency of HFE in all populations. We now know that HHC is the most common genetically transferred disease among white persons.

Within the same year as the gene discovery, the U.S. Centers for Disease Control and Prevention (CDC) surveyed nearly 3,000 individuals diagnosed with hemochromatosis. An impressive 80 percent, or 2,851 individuals, responded to the survey. Results were quite revealing and rather astonishing. From the 2,851 respondents, it was learned that 67 percent of those with symptoms had been given multiple, various diagnoses prior to receiving the proper diagnosis of hemochromatosis. Among the misdiagnoses were arthritis, gallbladder or liver disease, stomach disorders, hormonal deficiencies, psychiatric disorders, and diabetes. These patients indeed had these conditions, but their true underlying cause was being missed.

The average age of patients surveyed was forty-one. Of those who reported symptoms: 75 percent experienced chronic fatigue, 75 percent had joint pain, 58 percent reported a loss of libido, or loss of interest in sex, 44 percent had skin color changes, 41 percent experienced heart irregularities, and 35 percent reported abdominal pain. Thirty percent had no symptoms. Seventeen percent had been found anemic and were prescribed iron supplements, after being misdiagnosed with iron deficiency. It is still not widely recognized that iron overload can cause anemia, just as iron deficiency can; the mechanisms are quite

> ". . . MORE THAN 90% OF CLINICALLY DIAGNOSED HAEMOCHROMATOSIS PATIENTS OF EUROPEAN HERITAGE ARE HOMOZYGOTES FOR THE C282Y MUTATION OF THE HFE GENE."
>
> —*IRON2000 USA Scientific Conference, and EASL International Consensus Conference on HC* Journal of Hepatology *2000*

different, however! Another 18 percent reported they had taken iron supplements for their health. The most disturbing finding, however, was that the average length of time before proper diagnosis was reached was nine and a half years, after having seen at least three different physicians.

Even though the CDC survey included a relatively small sample of the U.S. population, the survey results documented many similarities among patients with hemochromatosis. The CDC's efforts gave hope to many patients who had been trying for years to bring attention to the disorder. Patients who participated in focus groups felt that the results of the survey allowed a closer look and a better understanding of a hemochromatosis patient profile.

Most physicians learned in medical school that hemochromatosis was rare, an older man's disease. As clinicians, they were trained how to recognize and treat diabetes, arthritis, heart trouble, liver disease, depression, infertility, and sexual dysfunction. A doctor might tell a patient that the cause of a disease is idiopathic (unknown), or genetic, and may offer nothing more. Eliminating symptoms, so the patient is relieved of pain or distress, seems a more reasonable goal than chasing a rare cause. Anyone who has had a severe headache that goes away with the right pain reliever has experienced the same sequence of events as a physician who is trying to heal a sick patient.

Still, it is difficult for patients with hemochromatosis to understand why some physicians respond with skepticism toward the disorder. HHC patients who are aware of prevalence studies feel these studies represent scientific proof that hereditary hemochromatosis is common. In 1996, when Mercator Labs made the worldwide announcement about the discovery of the HFE gene and its mutations, people with hereditary hemochromatosis thought an immediate change in perspective among physicians would follow. It did not. Scientists were ecstatic. They had the genetic key to unlock the door to numerous mysteries about hemochromatosis, but response from the medical community was lukewarm at best.

> "WHAT CAME THROUGH REPEATEDLY FROM PARTICIPANTS [OF THE FOCUS GROUPS] WAS THE LACK OF KNOWING ABOUT HHC AMONG PHYSICIANS."
>
> —*Betty Thomas, focus group participant and hemochromatosis patient*

Penetrance and Other Baffling Hemochromatosis Issues

For unknown reasons, hemochromatosis manifests differently among individual patients. Some patients with hemochromatosis get very ill, others not at all. Males with undetected HHC can die in their fifties of heart failure. Females with the disorder might not have cardiac symptoms until they reach their seventies. There are some people who have few symptoms, and others who have many. Even among family members who have the same HFE gene mutations, each person can display a different combination of symptoms and laboratory test results.

One sibling might have heart trouble and hormonal problems, another joint pain and diabetes, and yet another might have gallbladder and liver problems. One family member might have seriously elevated serum ferritin, while another has only somewhat elevated serum ferritin. Some respond to therapy without complications while others get worse.

Because almost all the symptoms of hemochromatosis have other, more common, explanations, the correct diagnosis is not always immediately apparent until a physician has become familiar with hemochromatosis. Otherwise, these seemingly unrelated combinations of symptoms and test results remain an unexplained phenomenon or are ascribed to some more common cause.

Geneticists use the word *penetrance* to describe this phenomenon of how a gene expresses itself in a person. A penetrance that varies and is less than 100 percent helps to perpetuate skepticism among physicians about how common hemochromatosis actually is.

2

Iron in Your Body

If you were asked to describe iron, how would you do it? You might say that iron is the second most common mineral on earth and is the stuff used to make magnets, barbells, nails, the rust stains in your bathtub, bridges and tall buildings, or your granny's skillet. Or you might add that iron is a pill you can take to remedy fatigue caused by anemia. You would be correct to some extent with any one of these descriptions of iron. However, you may not know that iron is a metal so essential that without it most life on this planet would cease to exist. Plants would wither and die; animals and human beings would suffocate.

Plants require iron to make chlorophyll. Plants, animals, and human beings require iron to make DNA, which encodes all life. Animals and humans also need iron to make hemoglobin, which delivers oxygen to the body; also, we need iron to make myoglobin in muscles. Myoglobin is a protein like hemoglobin, except that it is an oxygen storage protein contained in muscles of the body. We call upon the oxygen stored in myoglobin when we use our muscles to walk, run, climb, or move in any way.

On the other hand, iron can be so deadly that 450 milligrams can poison a small child. Too much iron absorbed from diet, injections, or repeated blood transfusion can accumulate to levels that "rust" vital organs and cause them to fail. Remember that streak of iron in the bathtub? That's rust or iron oxide; the same thing can be present in your liver, joints, pancreas, heart, brain, lungs, and skin if too much iron gets into your system.

So what is this magical but potentially lethal metal? Where does it come from, and how do we get it? Iron is a metallic element that is found in plants, animals, soil, meteorites, and rocks, including ones found on the surface of the moon. Here on earth, plants absorb iron through their root systems; animals eat these plants, and humans consume these plants and animals.

> # MYTH
>
> ***Iron is a***
> ***heavy metal***
> **INCORRECT**
>
> Iron is a micronutrient;
> heavy metals include
> lead, arsenic, mercury,
> cadmium, thallium,
> gold, and platinum.

Most of us can get sufficient amounts of iron from daily diets that include a moderate amount of meat. However, humans can get iron in other ways that might be harmful. We can inhale it in firsthand or secondhand tobacco smoke, take excessive amounts of supplemental iron, or we can receive iron by injection or blood transfusions. We can also overdo on alcohol consumption, which enhances the absorption of iron.

Some Forms of Iron Must Be Changed to Be Absorbed

Iron in Granny's skillet is elemental iron. This form of iron cannot be absorbed by the body; it must be oxidized or changed by being united with oxygen. Bound with oxygen, elemental iron becomes ferric oxide or common rust. The body cannot absorb iron in this form either. Iron must be changed into ferrous iron, which occurs when ferric oxide is exposed to an acidic environment. This is accomplished in the stomach when ferric oxide mixes with adequate hydrochloric acid (HCL, or stomach acid).

Iron Is Ready to Be Absorbed and Transported

Iron moves out of the stomach into the duodenum, the portion of the small intestine where the majority of absorption will take place. Ferrous iron is able to be absorbed in the duodenum. With the exception of another possible opportunity for a small amount of absorption that can take place later in the digestive system, all other iron will continue on to be excreted. Absorbed iron is grabbed by fingerlike projections called villi, which line the surface of the intestinal wall. Villi can pull iron into cells that then pass the metal into the bloodstream where it is met by a transport protein molecule called transferrin. Each molecule of transferrin can bind with and carry two atoms of iron.

Transported and Utilized
Scientists have been studying iron transport since the early 1940s. Two New York scientists, A. L. Schade and L. Caroline, noted an anti-infective agent in human plasma. They called it siderophilin; the name was later changed to transferrin. The term "siderophilin" also applies to lactoferrin. Transferrin and lactoferrin form a unique class of proteins. Transferrin remains the best-known transporter protein for iron, though candidate transport proteins are on the scientific horizon.

Lactoferrin is found in human secretions such as tears, perspiration, vaginal fluid, and mother's milk. It binds with iron, but lactoferrin is not considered a transporter of iron; instead, lactoferrin's role is entirely defense-related. Lactoferrin can withhold iron from invading microorganisms. However, H. pylori, a cause of gastic ulcer, actually seeks out lactoferrin-bound iron contained in the lining of the stomach. Lactoferrin-bound iron gives H. pylori its initial nourishment, enabling the microorganism to bore through the stomach wall, where it will then obtain iron directly from hemoglobin.

Some microorganisms are skilled in other ways in obtaining iron from human hosts. Staph, for example, can break open red blood cells and extract the iron it needs. Another pathogen, the protozoan that causes malaria, can get into the red blood cell to obtain iron necessary to thrive. And finally, there are bacteria, such as the one that causes tuberculosis, that grow best inside macrophages that are iron-loaded. Macrophages are white blood cells that protect us against disease; they scavenge for harmful invaders that enter our bloodstream. Iron-loaded macrophages are helpless to defend us against opportunistic infection and disease.

Transferrin is found in blood. Normally it is 25 to 35 percent saturated with the metal, but when there is too much iron for transferrin to carry, trouble can develop. Transferrin molecules that are heavily saturated lose the ability to tightly bind iron. Unbound or free iron is highly destructive and dangerous. Unbound iron can trigger free-radical activity, which can cause cell death and destroy DNA. Free iron can also provide nourishment for pathogens such as Yersinia, Listeria, and Vibrio bacteria. These bacteria are harmless for people with normal iron levels, but when transferrin is highly saturated with iron, Yersinia, Listeria and Vibrio (contained in raw shellfish such as oysters) can be deadly.

When working normally, transferrin binds to iron and transports it to all tissues, vital organs, and bone marrow so that normal metabolism, DNA synthesis, and red blood cell production can take place. Current research has discovered that transferrin does not work completely alone in the transport of iron. Ceruloplasmin, a protein that binds with copper, is involved in iron transport. Iron needs adequate amounts of copper to reach some of its intended destinations, including the brain.

A protein transporter called divalent metal transport ions (DMTI) recently was observed in mice and rats to have an iron-binding and transport ability. DMTI activity, however, seems to occur at a different phase of iron's journey. Some scientists theorize that there is more than one pathway through which iron is transported. They speculate that since there are different types of iron (plant, animal), perhaps there is more than one pathway available for transport. In any event, absorbed iron that is not needed for metabolism, production of DNA, or hemoglobin synthesis is placed within cells as ferritin.

Contained for Future Use or to Protect Us

Ferritin is a protein that is produced by nearly every cell of the body. It is a huge molecule; one ferritin molecule alone can hold up to 4,500 atoms of iron. Ferritin serves as a containment device for the metal when iron is in ample quantity or when iron has the potential to be harmful to one's health. Elevated serum ferritin can be an indicator that disease, or potential disease-causing factors, may be present.

Like transferrin, ferritin can also become unstable and ineffective. Think of ferritin like a big sink; when this sink gets full, ferritin and its iron can be changed into a precipitate called hemosiderin.

Hemosiderin can accumulate in cells of the heart, liver, lungs, pancreas, and other organs, restricting their ability to function.

For example, when beta cells (insulin-producing cells of the pancreas) are loaded with hemosiderin, these cells become unable to produce or store adequate amounts of the hormone insulin, which results in diabetes.

Scientists can obtain small amounts of tissue with a needle biopsy, stain it, and see hemosiderin in cells. For hemosiderin to be removed, it must be placed back into ferritin, which then may release the metal to form hemoglobin. The latter can be removed by phlebotomy, which is continued until iron deficiency is achieved in the patient.

Clearly, excessive accumulation of iron endangers health, but iron can be harmful to a person's health in another way.

Oxidative Stress or Free Radical Activity
Iron can reduce or change oxygen in two ways: As a chemical component of heme in hemoglobin iron is capable of carrying oxygen throughout the body. Behaving in this way, iron is a lifesaver. However, "free" or unbound iron can produce free radicals, which may damage cells.

Free radicals (FR) are normal byproducts of human metabolism as oxygen is utilized. FRs are atoms or groups of atoms that have at least one unpaired electron. More stable and less reactive chemical structures as a rule have their electrons all paired to one another. Free radicals are on the hunt for an additional electron and are highly reactive with other chemicals in the body.

Programmed from its creation to find its missing part, the FR steals electrons from anywhere in the body to make up for its missing partner. The free radical can steal from any cell in any organ, including the heart, pancreas, brain, liver, joints, etc. Free radicals can also change the structure of DNA. Once DNA is changed or mutated, it is passed on in this mutated form for all future generations. The free radical doesn't care about preserving a human cell or DNA, it only wants its missing part. Ravaged atoms within the cell are now also missing a part, which creates a chain reaction unleashing free-radical activity at increasing speed.

Examples of oxidation include rotting foods, rust you might see on a car or lawn furniture. Often, as in the case of the oxidation of fats, this sets off chain reactions, with one radical causing the destruction of hundreds or thousands of previously normal molecules. Iron-triggered free-radical activity can contribute to liver disease, pancreatic "burn out" (type II diabetes), joint disease, heart disease, neurological problems, and acceleration of aging, to name a few of the consequences of oxidative stress on the body.

Antioxidants protect the body from free-radical damage. An antioxidant donates or gives up the sought-after electron to a free radical and renders it harmless. Our bodies contain antioxidants obtained from fresh fruits and vegetables in our diets. When our diets lack fresh fruits and vegetables or are high in fats and sugars we can have an overabundance of free-radical activity.

Taking antioxidants, however, is not enough for those with elevated iron levels. Removing excess iron from the body with therapeutic phlebotomy or simple blood donation is the only way to diminish the risk of disease for these individuals.

Iron That Is Not Absorbed

For those with normal iron metabolism, unabsorbed iron, about 90 percent of iron ingested through diet, is taken up by specific cells in the intestinal tract called enterocytes. These cells become engorged with iron, die, drop off, and are excreted in feces. The portion of iron that gets absorbed is in the form of heme from the meat one consumes, non-heme from the plants we eat, and inorganic or chelated iron from supplements and food additives.

Resounding Airport Metal Detectors—A Personal Experience

Navy Master Chief Arthur Callahan did not know what it meant to walk through the Memphis airport metal detector without causing the annoying, and somewhat embarrassing, high-pitched squeal of the security equipment. Arthur dutifully dumped cigarette lighters, pocket change, his watch and anything else metal onto the tray provided by the attendant. His uniform prompted airport personnel to ask if he had any shrapnel or metal plates in his body. "Nope," Arthur answered as the attendant concluded a full-body examination with a hand-held wand.

> "WHAT SETS OFF AIRPORT METAL DETECTORS IS THE METAL ITSELF. IRON IS AFTER ALL, A METAL."
>
> —*Eugene Weinberg, Ph.D., Professor of Microbiology, Indiana University, Iron Disorders Institute Scientific Advisory Board Member*

It would be another ten years before Arthur would get an explanation of why metal detectors resounded as he passed through their sensors. His iron-overload condition would be revealed as a result of his 2,800 ferritin and 70 percent saturation. Today, Arthur is sufficiently de-ironed to expect "peace and quiet" when he departs from the same Memphis airport.

How Much Iron Is in the Body?
Males have about 4 grams of iron in their body, females about 3.5 grams; children will usually have 3 grams or less. These 3–4 grams are distributed throughout the body in hemoglobin, tissues, muscles, bone marrow, enzymes, ferritin, hemosiderin, and transport in plasma.

The greatest portion of iron in a normal human being is in hemoglobin. Except in cases of great blood loss, pregnancy, or growth spurts, where larger amounts of iron are required, our bodies only need about 1 to 1.5 milligrams of iron per day to replace what is lost. Normal daily excretion of iron through urine, vaginal fluid, sweat, feces, and tears totals about 1–1.5 milligrams, or

IRON DISTRIBUTION	males 4 grams females 3.5 grams children 3 grams
hemoglobin	70%
myoglobin and enzymes	15%
ferritin	14%
transit in serum	1%

the equivalent of what most of us require per day to function normally. Tiny amounts of iron can also be lost because of blood loss that can occur when medicines such as aspirin are used regularly.

Our Natural Iron Regulatory Mechanisms and Recommended Dietary Allowances
The average daily diet of an American vegetarian contains about 6–10 milligrams (mgs) of iron. Other American daily diets are reported to contain up to 23.5 milligrams of iron; these diets contain meat with most meals. Iron is not easily absorbed unless one has a metabolic disorder associated with iron loading like hemochromatosis.

Some nutrients that are not easily absorbed, such as iron, are given higher RDAs in an attempt to assure that adequate amounts of the essential nutrient are ingested within the course of a day. Attempts to meet daily requirements by ingesting quantities of iron that exceed daily need is, for many, a waste of time, money, and resource. Humans have a natural regulatory mechanism that controls the amount of iron absorbed based on needs. Therefore, when we take in large amounts of supplemental iron, this regulatory mechanism will signal the body to absorb less of the metal. Continuing to take large doses of unneeded iron will simply cause stomach and intestinal discomfort without added benefit.

1989 Recommended Dietary Allowance (RDA) for Iron and the Proportion of Americans Having Diets Meeting 100% of the RDA for Iron, 1994-1996		
Age (In Years)	1989 RDA (mg/day)	Proportion of Americans Meeting 100% of the RDA of Iron (%) from 1994-1996
FEMALES AND MALES		
<1	6-10	87.9[§]
1-2	10	43.9
3-5	10	61.7
FEMALES ONLY		
6-11	10	60.9
12-19	15	27.7
20-29	15	25.9
30-39	15	26.6
40-49	15	22.1
50-59	10	55.2
60-69	10	59.3
≥70	10	59.2
MALES ONLY		
6-11	10	79.8
12-19	12	83.1
20-29	10	86.9
30-39	10	88.9
40-49	10	85.9
50-59	10	83.8
60-69	10	85.5
≥70	10	78.5

Drs. Fariba Roughead and Janet Hunt, of the USDA Grand Forks Human Nutrition Research Center, conducted a study of the effects of iron supplements on the body's control of iron absorption. In a randomized, placebo-controlled trial, heme and non-heme iron absorption by healthy men and women were measured from a test meal containing a hamburger, potatoes, and a milk shake. These absorption measurements were made before and after a period of twelve weeks when the 57 participants were given 50 milligrams of supplemental iron or placebo daily while they consumed their usual diets.

Serum ferritin and fecal ferritin were measured during supplementation and for a period of six months after supplementation was discontinued. Volunteers who took iron supplements, even those with initial ferritin less than 21ng/mL, adapted to absorb less non-heme iron, but not less heme iron from meat.

Daily iron supplements caused these volunteers to absorb 36 percent less non-heme iron and 25% less total iron from food, and to have higher iron stores than those in the placebo group. The higher ferritin persisted for six months post-supplementation, except in individuals who had low iron stores at the beginning of the study. Since iron stores were greater after iron supplementation, Drs. Roughead and Hunt's study demonstrated that adaptation in absorption did not completely prevent differences in body iron stores.

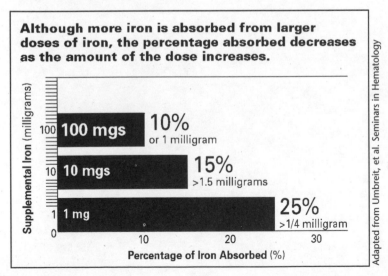

Although more iron is absorbed from larger doses of iron, the percentage absorbed decreases as the amount of the dose increases.

Supplemental Iron (milligrams)

100 **100 mgs**   **10%** or 1 milligram

10 **10 mgs**   **15%** >1.5 milligrams

1 **1 mg**   **25%** >1/4 milligram

Percentage of Iron Absorbed (%)

Adapted from Umbreit, et al. Seminars in Hematology

The adaptation to reduce iron absorption even in volunteers with low iron stores may indicate a localized control system to prevent excessive iron exposure of intestinal cells. The study is consistent with two systems at work, one that regulates how much iron we must absorb for normal function, and the iron withholding defense system, which protects us from nurturing harmful pathogens with excesses of iron we don't presently need.

3

Our One-Sided View of Iron

J. B. Williams Company, one of the smaller drug companies of the 1950s, needed a gimmick to sell one of its products, a multivitamin called Geritol. Instead of selling it for what it was, a nutritional supplement for iron deficiency, the company decided to sell it as a "quick fix" remedy for fatigue, a known symptom of iron deficiency anemia. Even though the medical community knew fatigue could be a symptom of any number of conditions, a large portion of the public did not. By using the prefix Geri, for geriatric, the company was pushing iron to one of the groups that need it least.

Courtesy of ClickArt

Though ads selling Geritol as a remedy for fatigue ran only six years, and were eventually banned in 1969 by the Federal Trade Commission, Americans were hooked. The Geritol success sensitized the nation to iron deficiency. No matter how objective a person might be, those incessant commercials had an effect. "Tired blood" and "My wife, I think I'll keep her" are phrases still familiar to millions of Americans some thirty years later.

With repeated claims that "Geritol contains twice the iron as a pound of calves' liver!" and the notion that "tired blood is iron-poor blood," it was only a matter of time before the medical community was influenced. Many physicians were prompted to write prescriptions for iron at the patient's first mention of fatigue. Though iron supplementation may be necessary in confirmed cases of iron deficiency anemia, it is not appropriate for those with iron loading disorders such as hemochromatosis where the number one complaint is "fatigue."

"OF 2,851 PEOPLE WITH HEMOCHROMATOSIS WHO RESPONDED TO THE SURVEY, 17 PERCENT HAD BEEN PRESCRIBED IRON SUPPLE-MENTS BY THEIR DOCTOR, AND ANOTHER 18 PERCENT REPORTED THEY HAD TAKEN IRON SUPPLEMENTS FOR THEIR HEALTH."

—*1996 Centers for Disease Control and Prevention HHC Patient Survey*

Iron deficiency anemia remains a worldwide health concern issue, but it is important to recognize that undiagnosed iron overload is also a major concern. An estimated 0.5 percent, or one million Americans, represent this subgroup of our population and are possibly being harmed by the supplemental iron contained in fortified food. Moreover, twenty-eight million persons, or about 10 percent of the U.S. population, are possible carriers of iron loading genes. It is now known that some of these carriers also absorb too much iron. Labeling of food products indicating the amount of iron content will help those who know they have abnormal iron metabolism. But what about the many who are unaware of their iron loading condition?

4

Iron Imbalances—Not Always What They Seem

Paula was ten years old when her doctor told her she was anemic and needed to take iron pills. Dr. Williams wanted to remove Paula's tonsils, but her anemia first had to be corrected. Since Paula's fifth birthday, tonsillitis was a frequent condition for her. This necessitated several rounds of penicillin. Paula wasn't looking forward to a tonsillectomy, but if it would help her fatigue and weakness enough to be with her friends, she would not mind having her tonsils removed. Attempting to get her hemoglobin level high enough for surgery, Paula ate iron-rich foods, and took a prescribed 325 milligrams of iron two times a day. Improving her hemoglobin consumed her summer. While her friends romped and splashed in community pools, Paula watched remotely, not wanting to expend too much energy. Her tonsils were removed during Christmas break, but her symptoms didn't improve.

On a surgical follow-up examination, Paula wondered how long she would have to take supplemental iron. She asked her doctor, who responded with, "How long do you intend to live?"

At age thirty-five Paula began having joint pain; she never seemed to have energy, and her colon was a constant source of trouble. Still, she dutifully responded to the local Red Cross blood center's call for blood donation. Instructed to continue her iron pills, she began donating blood in 1978 and continued to do so regularly until 1993. Elevated liver enzymes following a steroid injection prompted a letter from the Red Cross telling her she could no longer donate blood.

Two years later her joint pain worsened. Paula heard about a physician who knew a great deal about iron; she made her appointment. Dr. Adams measured her iron levels and because they were high he explained about iron overload. Diagnosed with suspect hemochromatosis, Paula knew the forty-two years of taking iron pills had been slowly poisoning her. Without thirteen years of regularly donating blood, which had kept her tissue iron levels in check, Paula's story would have had a possible lethal outcome. She speculates about the diagnosis of anemia when she was ten. Since hemoglobin can drop slightly when infection is present, Paula wonders if her constant tonsillitis was the real reason for her lower than normal hemoglobin.

Anemia of Chronic Disease
Anemia can also occur because of the presence of chronic disease, such as inflammatory conditions or infection. Anemia of chronic disease (ACD) is initially mild and will correct when the underlying disease is addressed with proper treatment. In ACD, hemoglobin levels will be slightly lower than normal but with elevated ferritin. ACD can be present in conditions ranging from something as common and simple as an ear infection to the early stages of tumor development. This mild anemia can also be a sign to investigate the presence of tumor development in diseases such as cancer of the prostate, colon, breast, ovaries, testes, lung, liver, or pancreas. Specific tests such as alpha-fetoprotein and ferritin can help determine whether tumor formation is underway, prompting an early diagnosis.

Iron deficiency anemia occurs when demands for iron exceed supplies available as a result of poor diet, growth spurts, pregnancy, and chronic blood loss including over-bleeding. Anemia also occurs as a result of problems of absorption, which can lead to vitamin and mineral deficiencies, causing problems of red blood cell production which can result in reduced hemoglobin production. Other causes of anemia include red blood cell destruction problems known as hemolytic anemia, inherited disorders that result in hemoglobin formation abnormalities such as thalassemia and sickle-cell anemia, alcohol consumption, some prescription and nonprescription medications, inhalation of toxic agents, inadequate production of the hormone erythropoietin, and kidney failure.

With so many conditions that result in anemia one can see how difficult it might be to pinpoint the underlying cause. Therapy to correct anemia cannot be safely begun until the reason for anemia is identified. A common assumption is that iron pills or iron injections are required to correct anemia. This may be true for confirmed cases where iron deficiency anemina is due to diet insufficiencies.

Supplemental iron is not appropriate for anemia caused by other factors. Iron supplementation might actually be harmful in cases of anemia of chronic disease, especially where disease is due to cancer or to infections such as pneumonia or malaria; these microbial pathogens require iron to thrive and will proliferate in an iron-rich environment, accelerating disease. Supplemental iron can impede treatment therapy for viral Hepatitis B or C, and AIDS, where response to therapy can be improved by lowering tissue iron levels. For these reasons, iron supplementation should never be taken without the supervision of a physician.

Iron Deficiency Anemia
The best-known and most common cause of anemia is iron deficiency. The Centers for Disease Control and Prevention estimates five million women in the United States are iron deficient. This condition, however, is not common in adult males—only one-tenth of those diagnosed with iron deficiency anemia (IDA) are men. A small but significant number of adult males receiving therapeutic phlebotomy report symptoms of IDA due to over-bleeding.

According to Drs. James Cook, Skikne, Lynch, and Reusser of Kansas University Medical College, an estimated 3 percent of children age six months to two years, 2.6 percent of premenopausal and 1.9 percent of postmenopausal females, and about two-tenths of 1 percent of males in the United States are iron deficient. In this estimate, about three million, rather than five million females, are iron deficient. This minor discrepancy occurs as a result of a difference in hemoglobin values used to establish anemia. In defining anemia, the CDC uses a slightly higher hemoglobin value than the values used by Drs. Cook, Skikne, Lynch, and Reusser.

Diet
Diets poor in variety or that lack adequate amounts of meat, such as vegetarian diets, can lead to iron deficiency anemia. Females and young children tend to eat less meat than men. Meat contains heme, which is highly bioavailable to the body; it is more easily absorbed than non-heme iron. Vegetables, nuts, grains, and fruits contain mostly non-heme iron.

Pregnancy and Iron Needs
Humans with normal iron metabolism have a natural regulatory mechanism that will assure adequate amounts of iron are absorbed, so long as sufficient amounts are consumed through diet. This mechanism has been observed in menstruating females who absorb up to 50 percent more iron during the days of menstruation than when not menstruating. In a British study of 12 pregnant women, iron absorbed from a normal diet was increased fivefold at 24 weeks of gestation and ninefold at 36 weeks as compared with the amount absorbed at the seventh week during the pregnancy.

For many decades, a large number of pregnant women have been advised to routinely take supplements of 25–65 milligrams (mgs) of iron daily, even without laboratory evidence of subnormal hemoglobin values. The routine procedure, even though it may be unnecessary, often is considered to be harmless and to have some unknown benefit. However, in 1993 a U.S. Preventive Service Task Force of the Office of Disease Prevention and Health Promotion, U.S. Public Health Service, carefully reviewed fifty published studies about iron supplementation. The task force concluded that controlled trials have failed to demonstrate that iron supplementation, or changes in hematologic indexes, actually improve clinical outcome for the mother or newborn. Additionally, the review found "no evidence that giving iron during pregnancy will reduce the incidence of childhood anemia or abnormal cognitive development."

There is agreement, however, that pregnant women who have subnormal hematologic values of 11 g/dL or less, and who are iron deficient, should take supplemental iron. Moreover, underlying conditions that might be responsible for low iron values such as malaria, hookworm, H. pylori, or other causes of internal bleeding should promptly be treated. Iron supplementation during this time is best monitored by a physician and discontinued once anemia is corrected, which will be evident in improved hemoglobin values.

High hemoglobin values have been reported by individuals with hemochromatosis. These elevated levels are usually associated with smoking or dehydration. Whether or not high tissue iron directly contributes to increased hemoglobin values is not known. Monitoring values during pregnancy and keeping levels within normal range can provide immeasurable health benefits. A few studies have examined the possibility that high as well as low hemoglobin values might be detrimental to the mother or fetus. In Wales, a study of 54,000 pregnancies found that prenatal mortality, low birthweight, and preterm birth were more common in women with hemoglobin values either less than 10.4 g/dL, or greater than 13.2 g/dL, than in women who had hemoglobin within the range of 10.5–13.1 g/dL. Similarly, in the U.S., a study of 22,000 pregnancies found that incidence of perinatal mortality was as much as twofold higher in women with hemoglobin values of 8 g/dL, and up to fivefold higher in women with hemoglobin values of 14 g/dL, than women with hemoglobin ranges of 9.0 g/dL to 13.0 g/dL. In the same study, incidence of low birthweight and neonatal prematurity were greater in women whose hemoglobin levels were less than 8.0 g/dL or higher than 14 g/dL.

In a November 23, 2000, *JAMA* (p. 2611) article, entitled "Maternal Hemoglobin Concentration During Pregnancy and Risk of Stillbirth," Dr. Olof Stephansson and his colleagues report that stillbirths nearly doubled in women whose hemoglobin values were 14.5 g/dL or higher. The report went on to state that anemia, or hemoglobin values less than 11.0 g/dL, was not significantly associated with risk of stillbirth.

Lactating Females
A well-established belief is that another time of high iron demand for females is during lactation. Though lactating females can be iron deficient, the cause is probably due to blood loss as a result of childbirth, and not necessarily because they need extra iron to nourish a newborn. Another reason for iron

deficiency during lactation is that during the third trimester, the mother sends a large quantity of iron to her developing offspring. If her diet is iron-poor at this time, she will experience iron deficiency anemia. Lactating mothers indeed require extra calories and adequate fluids to enable them to produce milk, but it is not necessarily true that they need supplemental iron.

Unless a new mother's hemoglobin values are below 11 g/dL, an iron-rich diet will likely provide sufficient amounts of iron for her and her newborn. Adding meat to the diet is a good way to get iron and to boost hemoglobin values. For women who cannot afford meat, such as those who live in developing countries, or who come from low-income families, iron-fortified foods and supplemental iron may be essential. Conversely, females who can afford meat, and who consume adequate amounts, along with other iron-rich foods, should not experience iron deficiency anemia. A health care provider can monitor hemoglobin values and diet to assure that the right balance of iron is maintained.

Growth Spurts

Growth spurts generate an increased need for iron. This great demand triggers a signal for the body to increase the amount of iron absorbed. Besides in utero, major growth spurts occur in infancy, continuing into and through early childhood, adolescence, and puberty. Inadequate supplies of iron or improperly distributed iron during this time can result in delayed maturation, slowed mental development, and short stature. Since the brain requires large amounts of the metal, some experts suspect iron imbalances may be contributing to childhood disorders such as emotional outbursts and attention deficit disorder. Scientists such as James Connor, Professor of Anatomy and Neuroscience, University of Pennsylvania, Vice-Chair of the George M. Leader Alzheimer's Research Institute and Scientific Advisory Board Member, are investigating how iron in the brain is transported and distributed. Dr. Connor believes that the hemochromatotic brain may actually be iron deficient because of the maldistribution of the metal.

The First Years of Life

Newborns have a great need for iron. This need is reflected in a naturally high transferrin saturation percentage and high serum ferritin values that occur in the first few months of life. Elevated levels of iron represent the need for the metal and are not an indication of iron overload unless their levels exceed the normal range for their age and gender. Newborns and young infants have different normal ranges for iron from adults. Only a qualified pediatrician should make decisions about an infant's iron status and appropriate therapy to assure iron balance.

	TIBC	Serum Iron	Ferritin
Newborn	130-275 mg/dL	100-250 mcg/dL	
Age 1-30 days			6-400 ng/mL
Age 1-6 months			6-410 ng/mL
Infant (age 7-12 months)	220-400 mg/dL	40-100 mcg/dL	60-80 ng/mL
Child (1-5 years of age)	220-400 mg/dL	50-120 mcg/dL	6-24 ng/mL

Breastfeeding is the easiest and best approach to iron balance in infants. Though breast milk appears to be low in iron, it is actually normal. Mother's milk contains a perfect and unique form of iron, which is bound to lactoferrin, a siderophilin (binding-molecule) that provides that the iron contained in breast milk will be highly bioavailable to the infant.

According to the Department of Nutrition, University of California, Davis, "Breast feeding is sufficient to maintain adequate iron nutrition for most, if not all of the first year of life. Infants fed fortified formula containing 10–14 mg/L of iron are receiving as much as 24 times more iron per day than what breastfed infants consume."

Dr. Elina Hemminki, National Research Centre for Welfare and Health Services, Helsinki, Finland, an expert in infant growth and health, provides that when infants cannot be breastfed, ". . . infant formulas that contain as little as 0.5 mg/L of iron are sufficient to meet daily demands."

Another point made in the California report is that "anemic women, and women taking iron supplements, have levels of iron in their milk that are similar to those of non-anemic women." This suggests that the amount of iron the breastfed infant receives is highly regulated by the mother's body. Studies have

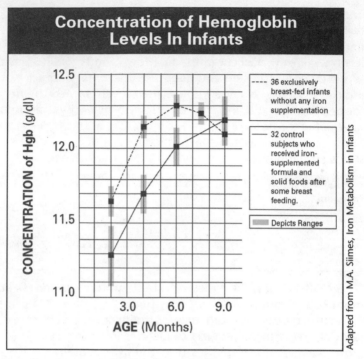

Concentration of Hemoglobin Levels In Infants

CONCENTRATION of Hgb (g/dl)

AGE (Months)

---- 36 exclusively breast-fed infants without any iron supplementation

— 32 control subjects who received iron-supplemented formula and solid foods after some breast feeding.

▮ Depicts Ranges

Adapted from M.A. Siimes, Iron Metabolism in Infants

shown that the amount of iron in breast milk cannot be increased by giving iron supplements to the mother.

At about the age of six to nine months, when an infant can be naturally weaned and introduced to cereals, a natural mild anemia in breastfed babies can be observed. During this period, babies with normal metabolism are not candidates for supplemental iron. Iron-rich diets can provide these children with adequate iron because their body will regulate what it needs to function. If anemia persists, however, or worsens, as observed by the pediatrician who is monitoring a child's hemoglobin and other values, further investigation to determine some other underlying cause for anemia is warranted.

Anemia in Youths
Anemia in young children, especially those younger than two, can be due to blood loss as a result of drinking cow's milk, intestinal parasites, or because of illness, especially when a fever

is present. When these conditions are corrected with appropriate treatment, hemoglobin levels should return to normal. Children with hemoglobin unresponsive to short-term iron supplementation may have a more serious condition, and should be seen by a pediatric hematologist or gastroenterologist.

Chronic Blood Loss Is a Common Reason for Iron Deficiency Anemia in Adults
For females who are menstruating, menorrhagia, or heavy periods, can result in as much as one cup of blood per period. One cup contains about 125 milligrams of iron. Prolonged heavy bleeding, where the duration might be as long as two weeks, may eventually lead to anemia if the loss is not offset with increased iron intake. Chronic blood loss can also occur from peptic ulcers, gastritis, and cancers of the gastrointestinal tract.

Acute blood loss can also happen as a result of trauma or surgery; whole blood transfusion is generally used therapeutically in these cases. Blood loss can also result from taking certain medications, such as those used to relieve arthritic pain.

> "HEMOGLOBIN VALUE IS ONE GOOD WAY TO DETECT THE PRESENCE OF ANEMIA. SERUM TRANSFERRIN RECEPTOR IS A GOOD WAY TO DETECT THE *CAUSE* OF ANEMIA. SERUM TRANSFERRIN RECEPTOR IS NOT AFFECTED BY INFLAMMATION OR INFECTION AND THEREFORE CAN DETECT THE DIFFERENCE BETWEEN IRON DEFICIENCY ANEMIA, ANEMIA OF CHRONIC DISEASE, AND IRON OVERLOAD."
>
> *—Dr. Barry Skikne,*
> *Kansas University Medical Center,*
> *Iron Disorders Institute Scientific*
> *Advisory Board Member*

Anemia in Adult Males
In males, iron deficiency anemia could be due to a vegetarian diet, but IDA in males is more often due to blood loss caused by internal bleeding. Common causes of blood loss include stomach ulcers caused by H. pylori, colon polyps, and bleeding hemorrhoids. Liver disease and bleeding esophageal varices are also causes of internal blood loss, but are not so common.

Emerging as a cause of blood loss that can result in iron deficiency anemia is over-bleeding during treatment for hemochromatosis/iron overload. With some of these conditions, oral iron supplementation or whole blood transfusion may become necessary to address an acute and life-threatening situation. For males who consume a diet that includes adequate amounts of meat, once acute blood loss has been corrected, routine supplementation with iron should not be necessary.

Absorption

Impaired absorption is another common cause of iron deficiency anemia. Insufficient hydrochloric acid (stomach acid), surgical removal of portions of the intestine, and gastrointestinal conditions such as Crohn's disease, can affect absorption. Lack of vitamin B_{12} can also have an effect on absorption of iron. B_{12} deficiencies lead to pernicious anemia, and B_{12} shots must be given regularly to provide the necessary amounts of this vital nutrient.

Experts in iron deficiency anemia such as Drs. Cook, Flowers, Skikne, and Baynes of Kansas University Medical Center,

Comparing test results of anemia of chronic disease (ACD), iron deficiency anemia (IDA) and iron overload (IO)			
	ACD	**IDA**	**IO**
hemoglobin (g/dL)	9-10	<10.5	normal
serum iron	decreased	decreased	increased
TIBC	decreased	increased	decreased
serum ferritin	increased	decreased	increased
TS%	decreased	decreased	increased
erythropoietin	inadequate	adequate	adequate
MCH/MCV	slightly decreased	decreased	normal
white blood cell	variable	normal	normal
red blood cell	decreased	normal	normal
serum transferrin receptor	normal	increased	normal/decreased
transferrin iron saturation percentage (TS%) mean corpuscular volume (MCV) total iron binding capacity (TIBC) mean corpuscular hemoglobin (MCH)			

determined that the serum transferrin receptor (sTfR) is a better way to diagnose true cases of iron deficiency anemia, when other chronic disorders exist. Serum transferrin receptor is not compromised by factors that affect ferritin. Furthermore, sTfR is sensitive enough to identify those mildly anemic or who are subclinically iron deficient. Subclinical cases are usually not identified until symptoms manifest.

Individuals with progressive iron deficiency initially experience depletion of iron storage (ferritin). Next, depletion of functional iron (hemoglobin) occurs. The sTfR is elevated between these phases even before hemoglobin drops below normal.

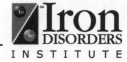

PART TWO

Detecting and Diagnosing Hemochromatosis

". . . HEMOCHROMATOSIS IS EASY TO DIAGNOSE WHEN YOU KNOW WHAT YOU'RE LOOKING FOR . . ."

—*Joseph A. De Stefano, M.D.,*
IRON2000 USA Patient Conference,
Greenville, South Carolina

5

Why Some Doctors Miss the Diagnosis of Hemochromatosis

Sick patients go to the doctor to get well. It's that simple. Getting the proper diagnosis, however, is not so simple. The process of diagnosis is complex, filled with twists and turns. A physician can see a patient with multiple symptoms of joint pain, headache, depression, heart arrhythmia, abdominal pain, and loss of libido and go in any number of directions for diagnosis. It is highly unlikely hemochromatosis will be the first condition that occurs to most physicians.

Thirty-year-old Brad went to his physician because of joint pain and chronic fatigue. He is often thirsty and has dry mouth. His parents are C282Y heterozygotes or carriers for hemochromatosis, but Brad isn't aware of this. His parents have been relatively healthy, and they are unaware they carry a potentially life-threatening genetic mutation. Brad has inherited one mutation from his dad and one from his mom, making him a C282Y homozygote—but he knows nothing about HFE and its mutations. Neither does his physician.

Brad's chances of being a homozygote are one in four, or 25 percent. His brothers and sister also have a 25 percent chance of being a homozygote, and a 25 percent chance being normal—no mutations, or a 50 percent chance of being a carrier themselves. Many carriers of the HFE mutation do not manifest symptoms—though there are some who do. Possibly these individuals possess other contributing genetic abnormalities not yet identified.

Brad's family history will offer few clues. When his physician hears nothing out of the ordinary by way of disease in his parents or siblings, he asks Brad about his grandparents. Brad remarks, "Oh yes, my grandmother had diabetes," which adds to the potential for misdiagnosis. His physician orders a blood glucose level because of the symptom of frequent thirst and family history of diabetes, and a rheumatoid factor test because of Brad's complaint of joint pain. Blood work reveals slightly elevated glucose and is negative for rheumatoid arthritis.

> "OF DIAGNOSED PARTICIPANTS WHO WERE HAVING SYMPTOMS, 67 PERCENT REPORTED THEY WERE DIAGNOSED FIRST WITH ARTHRITIS, LIVER/GALLBLADDER DISEASE, STOMACH DISORDERS, HORMONAL DEFICIENCIES, PSYCHIATRIC PROBLEMS, OR DIABETES BEFORE BEING PROPERLY DIAGNOSED WITH HEMOCHROMATOSIS."
>
> —*1996 CDC HHC Patient Survey*

Since diabetes is common, and after all, the patient's grandmother had diabetes, and he is symptomatic of the condition, Brad's physician makes the diagnosis of diabetes and misses the underlying cause, hemochromatosis. Brad is instructed to take an over-the-counter pain reliever for the joint pain, which his physician thinks is stress related. He gives Brad a prescription drug for glucose control, a copy of a diet, and tells him to reduce the stress in his life. He tells Brad that his sugar levels can be controlled through diet and medication, but if problems persist, he will make arrangements for Brad to see an endocrinologist, a physician who specializes in diabetes.

While Brad struggles to adhere to his diabetes diet, other conditions advance unchecked. Iron proceeds to accumulate in Brad's vital organs. Unbeknownst to him, liver cirrhosis has begun and his heart is being damaged irreversibly. His lungs are becoming diseased because he is a smoker, and essential glands such as his pituitary and thyroid are filling with iron, leaving him impotent and depressed. To round things off, Brad is beginning to lose body hair, but it is the loss of hair on his head that bothers him most.

He calls his family doctor and asks for that referral to the endocrinologist. Two months later, he gets his moment with the specialist, where he complains that the diabetes must be out of control. He has lost his libido (sex drive) and admits to being impotent. He complains about his hair loss and remarks that his fatigue is worse.

His endocrinologist tells Brad his symptoms are probably not related to diabetes, and that he suspects hypothyroidism; he tests Brad's thyroid function. The endocrinologist runs several other tests as well, including blood glucose. When test results confirm he has an underactive thyroid, Brad is relieved. Hair loss, chronic fatigue, and loss of interest in sex are symptoms associated with hypothyroidism. His doctor solves yet another mystery and prescribes thyroid hormone replacement therapy for Brad.

Modest improvement by way of increased energy and desire for sex fools Brad into thinking his problems are over; unfortunately, they are silently getting worse. Within weeks, Brad's fatigue returns. His libido begins to fade, and he develops abdominal pain, shortness of breath, chest pain, and notices his heart beats irregularly.

The endocrinologist cannot help; so, Brad calls his family doctor and is given a referral to a cardiologist for the heart trouble, and a gastroenterologist for the abdominal pain. Brad now tries to decide which doctor to see first. If he selects the gastroenterologist, he might receive the correct diagnosis of hemochromatosis. But fearing a heart attack, Brad contacts the cardiologist. Because Brad complains of chest pains, he gets an appointment right away.

The cardiologist gives Brad what seems a very thorough physical exam, complete with stress test, blood work, and EKG. Brad experiences no heart arrhythmia during this exam. "These things never seem to take place when a doctor is in the room," comments Brad. His EKG is normal, but because he is slightly overweight, the cardiologist gives him a low-fat diet and an exercise program of daily walking.

Brad tries faithfully to follow his new diet and exercise program. But ten days into his new routine, profound fatigue overpowers him. His motivation evaporates. He musters the strength to contact the gastroenterologist. He is so discouraged at this point that when the scheduling nurse asks if he prefers a morning or afternoon appointment, Brad hisses in response, "I don't give a damn! Just give me anything!" By now he is a physical and emotional wreck. His skin has darkened. Brad appears to have a tan, though he has not been in the sun. There are dark lines in the creases of his hands and dark circles under his eyes. He is still in pain; his head is pounding. He is depressed, over-weight, short of breath, and still having irregular heartbeats. He is impotent, has no interest in sex, and he watches in horror as far too many clumps of his hair swirl down the bathtub drain.

For some patients with hemochromatosis, Brad's story sounds all too familiar. False assumption can set a patient up for a series of misdiagnoses, possible mistreatment, and a seemingly unending cycle of symptoms-treatment-temporary relief-new symptoms-another diagnosis and so on.

Physicians are motivated to get a sick patient well—to stop the pain or problem that can be observed. It may never occur to them to check for a possible cause of these symptoms: hemochromatosis, a common genetic disorder of iron metabolism.

Fortunately for Brad, he finally sees a gastroenterologist who is familiar with hemochromatosis. After apologizing profusely to the scheduling nurse for his outburst on the phone, Brad's trans-ferrin iron saturation percentage, serum ferritin, and liver enzymes are measured. The gastroenterologist suspects Brad's symptoms to be related to hereditary human hemochromatosis (HHC). He notes that Brad's liver is enlarged (hepatomegaly). His fasting serum ferritin is over 3,000, his saturation is 97 percent, his liver enzymes are mildly elevated, and he is told he needs a liver biopsy to confirm diagnosis.

Though Brad undergoes a liver biopsy, this procedure was not necessary to diagnose hemochromatosis. His biopsy was, however, appropriate to determine the extent of liver damage. Brad's cirrhosis was clearly shown by the biopsy. His good news was that he did not have liver cancer. What his doctor did not tell him is that statisti-cally, when a diagnosis of hemochromatosis is made after cirrhosis has developed, the chance that the patient will develop liver cancer increases two hundredfold.

> "OF 2,845 PARTICIPATING HHC PATIENTS, 554 WERE DIAGNOSED BECAUSE DIAGNOSIS OF A FAMILY MEMBER LED THEM TO GET TESTED."
> —1996 CDC HHC Patient Survey

Another way Brad could have been diagnosed is by genetic testing; later, he opts to do this. It is no surprise that he is a C282Y homozygote. Brad immediately begins calling his siblings. One brother refuses genetic testing, fearing he would lose his job. Another brother is tested right away and is also a C282Y homozygote. His sister is considering genetic testing.

Brad starts therapeutic phlebotomy, and becomes successfully de-ironed. Some of his symptoms improve, some worsen, but at least he knows the cause of his years of pain and suffering. It has a name: hemochromatosis.

> "SYMPTOMS WERE EXPERIENCED AN AVERAGE OF 9 1/2 YEARS AND MORE THAN THREE PHYSICIANS WERE CONSULTED BEFORE PROPER DIAGNOSIS OF HHC WAS MADE."
>
> —*1996 CDC HHC Patient Survey*

Brad goes back to his family physician to share what he has learned. He carries with him some printed materials that explain how two simple tests, transferrin iron saturation percentage and serum ferritin, would have likely resulted in the proper diagnosis. Brad's medical journey and final discovery spanned eleven years and involved four physicians.

6

How Do I Know
If I Have Iron Overload?

There are more than 1,300 known metabolic disorders; hemochromatosis is one of them. Many of these disorders share similar symptoms with other conditions, which makes disorders of metabolism some of the most baffling and difficult to diagnose. A metabolic disorder exists because of defects somewhere in the body's production of energy. This process includes a complex series of events, involving the presence of specific enzymes, genes, blood proteins, hormones, vitamins, electrolytes, water, and minerals, such as iron, copper, zinc, and calcium. Further, normal metabolism requires the individual's ability to use these components, which involves absorption, transport, and synthesis. One abnormality, one missing enzyme, or one defect anywhere in the process, can disrupt normal metabolism.

In hereditary human hemochromatosis, some scientists believe that because HHC is an inherited condition, the error of iron metabolism occurs in more than one process and in more than one organ system. DNA is in every cell of the body. When a gene is mutated or flawed, its message is flawed throughout the entire human system. Therefore, the wrong message could take place anywhere within the iron regulatory and utilization process, creating several different symptom and test result combinations.

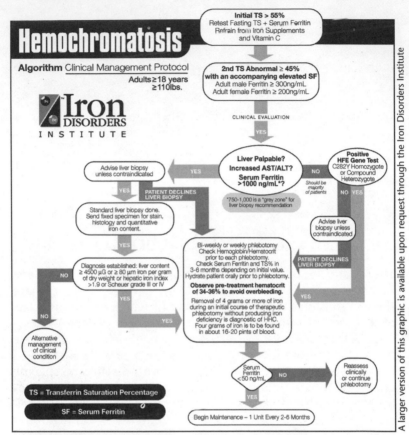

Contributions to the Hemochromatosis Algorithm made by Dr. Alex Hover, St. John's Regional Health System, U.S. Centers for Disease Control and Prevention, and Iron Disorders Institute Scientific Advisory Board

Diagnosis of iron overload begins with an elevated transferrin iron saturation percentage greater than 55 percent. Normal range for transferrin iron saturation percentage is 25–35 percent. Transferrin iron saturation percentage is a calculation derived from serum iron values divided by total iron binding capacity (TIBC) multiplied by one hundred.

An elevated transferrin iron saturation percentage greater than 55 percent should be followed by a second fasting saturation percentage and a serum ferritin. Fasting involves nothing by mouth after midnight or prior to blood work. Also, a patient should discontinue any vitamin supplements that contain great amounts of vitamin C, A, or iron, which can affect the result of the tests. Further, patients should cut back on sugary fruit juices, and drink ample water—two liters per day for an adult, one liter per day for a teen or adolescent.

Fasting transferrin iron saturation percentage and serum ferritin both will be elevated if excessive tissue iron is present.

LAB TEST RESULTS	Hemoglobin	Hematocrit	Ferritin	Transferrin Iron Saturation Percentage
Iron Overload	NORMAL 12-17 g/dL	NORMAL 36-42%	Elevated	Greater than 45%
Iron Deficiency Anemia	LOW	LOW	Less than 15 ng/mL	Less than 15%

Important Ferritin Reference Ranges		
ferritin	Adult Males	Adult Females
Normal Range	up to 300ng/mL	up to 200ng/mL
In treatment*	below 100ng/mL	below 100ng/mL
Ideal maintenance	25-75ng/mL	25-75ng/mL
Adolescents, Juveniles, Infants & Newborns of normal height and weight for their age and gender		
Male ages 10-19	23-70ng/mL	Infants 7-12 months 60-80ng/mL
Female ages 10-19	6-40ng/mL	Newborn 1-6 months 6-41ng/mL
Children ages 6-9	10-55ng/mL	Newborn 1-30 days 6-400ng/mL
Children ages 1-5	6-24ng/mL	

Elevated serum iron can be an indicator that hemochromatosis is present, but serum iron alone is not a reliable way to determine excessive tissue iron. Serum iron is influenced by many factors, such as time of day. Serum ferritin also can be unreliable. Ferritin is an acute phase reactant which means it is affected by any kind of inflammatory process. Inflammation can occur as a result of taking certain medications, such as hormone replacement therapy, and in the presence of chronic diseases, such as cancer, viral hepatitis, and liver disease.

A physical examination to check for liver or spleen inflammation is important. If either is palpable (physician can feel it with touch), liver biopsy may be indicated.

iron panel	IRON PANEL TESTS					
	Serum Iron	Serum Ferritin	Transferrin Iron Saturation Percentage	Total Iron Binding Capacity (TIBC)	Transferrin	Serum Transferrin Receptor
Hemochromatosis	↑	↑	↑	↓	↓	NORMAL TO LOW
Iron Deficiency Anemia	↓	↓	↓	↑	↑	HIGH
Sideroblastic Anemia	↑	↑	↑	↓	↓	NORMAL TO HIGH
Thalassemia	↑	↑	↑	↓	↓	HIGH
Porphyria Cutanea Tarda	↑	↑	↑	↓	↓	NORMAL
Anemia of Chronic Disease (ACD)	↓	↑ OR NORMAL	↓	↓	↓	NORMAL
African siderosis	↑	↑	↑	↓	↓	NORMAL TO LOW

Liver Biopsy

Diagnosis of hemochromatosis with liver biopsy, prior to 1998, was the only method recognized as reliable by physicians. This procedure is generally performed by a gastroenterologist and other specialists trained to do liver biopsy, including radiologists, general surgeons, and surgical oncologists.

Results are read by a pathologist, who dries and weighs the specimen. This will provide the pathologist with information needed to calculate a hepatic index, or the amount of iron concentration (expressed in micromoles of iron per gram of dry liver) in the liver, divided by the age of the patient in years. Hepatic iron greater than 80 mol/g or hepatic index greater than 1.9 confirms tissue iron overload. Pathologists can detect iron in another way. A sample of the tissue obtained from liver biopsy is stained with Prussian blue or Perl's stain. The sample is examined under a microscope where iron will appear as dark blue spots in liver cells on the pathologist's slide. Without stain, iron cannot be seen. Staining the tissue sample confirms the presence of iron; drying, weighing the tissue sample, then analyzing it for iron content confirms the amount of iron contained in the organ biopsied.

Liver Biopsy Experiences Vary
Two sisters, Andrea and Liz, lived about nine hundred miles apart. Both received a diagnosis of suspected hemochromatosis within a month of one another. Each was told she needed a liver biopsy to confirm the diagnosis.

The older sister, Liz, had been reading about hemochromatosis and liver biopsy. When her

> "LIVER BIOPSY IS NO LONGER NECESSARY TO DIAGNOSE HEMOCHROMATOSIS."
> —*IRON2000 USA Scientific Conference*

family physician referred her to a gastroenterologist, Liz knew a great deal about the procedure. It was important to Liz that she find a physician who had performed the procedure often and with few complications. She located patients who had received liver biopsies and eventually found such a physician. Her biopsy was easy, no complications. She had no lasting discomfort. "I felt a slight sensation of pressure," Liz says. "My younger sister had a different experience. Though she had no extraordinary problems during the procedure, she told me two days later, she felt like she had been kicked by a mule."

When Karl was told he needed a liver biopsy to confirm diagnosis of hemochromatosis, he declined. Karl's brother had been diagnosed several months earlier, and the family had been reading extensively about HHC. Karl had no symptoms. His saturation percentage was 88 percent and his serum ferritin was 670 ng/mL. His liver enzymes were normal, and he had no inflammation, in either his liver or spleen.

Karl had learned through his reading that liver biopsy is not necessary to diagnose hemochromatosis. He read that liver biopsy is used to determine cirrhosis, or sometimes primary liver cancer, and is used as a prognostic aid. In this way a biopsy provides information about a patient's chances of survival or quality of life while disease is present. In the case of liver disease, a biopsy can detect how much iron has collected in the liver and the extent of cirrhosis, fibrosis, or the presence of cancer. Liver biopsy remains the only way to determine the extent of damage to the liver.

Drs. Guyader, Jacquelinet, Moirand, Turlin, Mendler, Chaperon, David, Brissot, Adams, and Deugnier, a team of French scientists, who are experts in iron metabolism, found that patients who are C282Y homozygotes whose serum ferritin is less than 1,000 ng/mL, who have no hepatomegaly (enlargement of the liver) and normal liver enzymes, have less than 1 percent chance of cirrhosis. Most patients will opt out of having a liver biopsy as a means of diagnosis, knowing there are other less invasive ways to diagnose hemochromatosis.

Options to Liver Biopsy for Diagnosis of Hemochromatosis
Today's physicians have several noninvasive and cost-effective ways to confirm diagnosis, such as quantitative phlebotomy, specialized MRI, and genetic testing. There are also situational opportunities where hemochromatosis might not be suspect, but proper diagnosis results because of these events, which can include abnormal test results, preexisting disease, and an informed patient.

> "MRI CANNOT BE STRESSED ENOUGH FOR PEOPLE WITH HEMOCHROMATOSIS."
>
> —*Dr. James Connor, Professor of Anatomy and Neuroscience, Pennsylvania State University and Iron Disorders Institute Scientific Adviser*

Specialized magnetic resonance imaging (MRI) can detect the presence of iron in organs such as the liver, heart, lungs, pancreas, and brain. An MRI can even detect iron in small glands such as the pituitary. Iron will appear as dark areas on the film. A trained radiologist will be able to distinguish the difference between darkness caused by a tumor and darkness caused by iron. Specialized MRI is emerging as a good, noninvasive way to confirm the presence of iron in all major organs of the body. An MRI, however, will expectedly be normal in persons when performed before sufficient time has passed for significant overload to occur.

MRI requires a fairly large piece of equipment. A patient must lie on a table, which slides automatically into a open, tunnel-like cylinder that is actually a magnet. Radio frequencies interact with the magnet, providing information to sensors. As signals pass through the body, these sensors detect them. An increase in liver iron decreases the intensity of a signal, resulting in a dark area on the x-ray film.

Quantitative Phlebotomy
In standard phlebotomy, about one pint or 450–500cc of blood are removed. This unit contains approximately 200–250 milligrams of iron. Quantitative phlebotomy is the technique where the total amount of iron ultimately removed is calculated to determine whether the total body iron load is increased. Four grams of iron are found in about 16–20 pints of blood. Individuals who have four grams or more of mobilizable iron by quantitative phlebotomy can be diagnosed as having iron overload. A conclusive diagnosis of hemochromatosis cannot be made in this way; but hemochromatosis can be highly suspect in such individuals. Genetic testing can be considered in these cases.

> "... THERE IS AMPLE EVIDENCE THAT C282Y/H63D HETEROZYGOTES ARE AT HIGH RISK OF DEVELOPING HEMOCHROMATOSIS."
> —*Iron2000 USA Scientific Conference John Feder, Ph.D., HFE Gene Discovery Team, Iron Disorders Institute Scientific Advisory Board Member*

Our example patient Karl, mentioned earlier, opted for quantitative phlebotomy over liver biopsy, and was eventually diagnosed with the genetic test.

Genetic Testing
Genetically testing a patient for the presence of C282Y and H63D mutations of HFE is a good noninvasive way to diagnose hereditary hemochromatosis. Read more about genetics in chapter nine.

> "MORE THAN 90 PERCENT OF THOSE DIAGNOSED WITH HEMOCHROMATOSIS WHO ARE OF NORTHERN EUROPEAN DESCENT ARE HOMOZYGOTES FOR THE C282Y MUTATION OF HFE."
> —*EASL International Consensus Conference on Haemochromatosis*, Journal of Hepatology *2000*

7

Clues That Can Lead
to Diagnosis

Sometimes unplanned events such as abnormal test results can lead to proper diagnosis. Elevated liver enzymes or elevated serum iron can prompt a physician to suspect hemochromatosis and confirm diagnosis with further testing. Prior to 1997, serum iron was included in routine blood panels such as the Executive Panel offered by LabCorp of America and its subsidiaries.

On November 25, 1996, San Diego Regional Laboratory of Allied Clinical Laboratories, Inc., pled guilty to submitting a false claim to Medicare and to the California Medicaid Program for unnecessary blood tests and was fined $5 million as a result. Allied was then owned by LabCorp, which agreed to pay $182 million to the Department of Health and Human Services Medicare/Medicaid Program to resolve the allegations.

The matter of overcharging came to the attention of California law enforcement officials after a doctor noticed that the laboratory he was using routinely did tests that he did not ask for directly. The inclusion of serum iron in these Executive Panels provided an unknown side benefit. Numerous people were properly diagnosed with hemochromatosis as a result of an elevated serum iron.

Unfortunately, changes in Health Care Finance Administration (HCFA) policy guidelines for reimbursement resulted in the removal of serum iron and serum ferritin from comprehensive blood panels because they were considered "unnecessary costs."

HCFA presumed that people were being tested unnecessarily, and that money from these extra tests was creating a windfall for some laboratories. Thus no reimbursement would be made for such tests unless a physician ordered them specifically to confirm diagnosis.

So in 1997, serum iron was removed from these panels along with other tests considered unnecessary, resulting in a complete upheaval of the diagnostic process. Individual tests now must be ordered by a physician as a result of diagnosis. In other words physicians had to know the diagnosis, and could only order those tests that would confirm diagnosis— actually the physician could order any number of tests, HCFA reimbursement guidelines, however, would only pay for those relative to the diagnosis.

> **DID YOU KNOW** ⁉️
>
> **Serum iron and serum ferritin were removed from panels as a result of Medicare guideline policy changes in an effort to reduce unnecessary charges.**

What was overlooked by HCFA policy decision-makers was that elevated serum iron had contributed·to the correct diagnosis of possibly as many as one-third of the people diagnosed with hemochromatosis during the years between 1990 and part of 1997. Some of these individuals had gone to their physician seeking a cause for symptoms; some went for routine physicals, and were diagnosed pre-symptomatically.

Preexisting Disease Conditions Offer Subtle Clues

When a patient mentions history of arthritis, diabetes, heart trouble or arrhythmia, liver problems, or previous experience with evaluated liver enzymes, especially mildly elevated liver enzymes, these can be clues to suspect hemochromatosis. Other conditions where hemochromatosis might be suspect include amenorrhea, anterior pituitary failure, diabetes type I and II, impotence and loss of libido, inappropriate increased skin pigmentation, infertility, liver cancer, and porphyria cutanea tarda (PCT).

> "ELEVATED SERUM IRON IS AMONG THE MOST COMMON REASONS GIVEN FOR HOW DIAGNOSIS OF HHC WAS OBTAINED."
>
> —*Iron Disorders Institute, Patient Services*

Listening to a Patient Can Bring About the Correct Diagnosis

"You don't need to be tested for hemochromatosis," Clara's physician remarked. "It's rare and it doesn't occur in women," he concluded and closed her file, which was several inches thick. Clara looked at her doctor, trying to remain civil. "Just humor me, and do the tests."

Clara had been searching for answers about her health for more than four years. Her extensive reading had led her to believe that she might have hemochromatosis. Her father had died at age fifty-nine of a sudden heart attack. He had other problems, which were not mentioned openly while he was alive. Clara's mother eventually admitted that Clara's father had often been depressed, and drank heavily, especially at bedtime. He had lost all interest in sex and was so exhausted he missed work frequently. She was ashamed to tell anyone that her husband was an alcoholic. Besides, he would often have emotional outbursts that worked well as a deterrent for telling anyone about his condition. She was shocked when he died of a heart attack; she thought his liver would fail long before his heart.

> "OVER 45 PERCENT OF THOSE WHO RESPONDED TO THE SURVEY WERE DIAGNOSED PRE-SYMPTOMATICALLY BECAUSE OF ABNORMAL LAB TESTS."
>
> —*U.S. Centers for Disease Control and Prevention 1996 HHC Patient Survey*

Clara wasn't certain that her father died of hemochromatosis, but her own personal battle with unresolved health issues made her think it could be possible. Besides, she rationalized, a saturation percentage test wasn't very expensive and if her suspicions were true, whatever the cost, it would be worth it.

Clara's saturation percentage was indeed elevated. Her repeat fasting saturation percentage was 48 percent, and her ferritin was 137 ng/mL, not high enough, according to her physician, to order a phlebotomy. She asked to be genetically tested, and was found to be a C282Y/H63D compound heterozygote.

Females are usually more persistent than males in the pursuit for health-related information. Males tend to consult or visit their doctors less often than females. According to the Pew Internet &

American Life Project, a research center created to take a comprehensive in-depth look at the social impact of the Internet, "Females are more likely to go online to look for medical and health information (61 percent for women vs. 47 percent for men)." Usually, these women are motivated by the illness of their husband, child, sibling, parent, or other close relative. Educated by information from medical libraries, the Merck Manual, the Internet, and patient advocacy groups, these women are determined to be heard.

According to Dr. Mark Princell, St. Francis Health System, Greenville, SC, "A self-educated patient can be a pleasure or a nightmare. When a patient obtains information from reliable resources, they come to us with a good basic understanding of their health condition. It makes our jobs easier."

In today's information age, patients are taking a more active role in their health. They are reading more and learning a lot about disease-causing conditions. Some are getting properly diagnosed earlier as a result of good solid investigation. However, no matter how well-read a patient might be, he or she is still medically untrained and may not be able to distinguish between safe or risky medicine.

The Internet can be an invaluable resource, but it is currently an information free-for-all. Patients are correct to seek information from this resource, but they need to know how to qualify what they download. Most doctors are appreciative of any new and breaking medical information. When cooperation exists between patient and physician, the patient gets the benefit of his or her doctor's years of medical training. Likely, the harmful information will be identified and discarded during such a cooperative exchange. Qualified physicians see several hundred patients a week—whereas, a patient is probably limited to his or her own family experience with illness. Disaster is in the making when a patient, emotionally charged from misinformation, challenges his or her physician to a medical duel.

One Misinformed Patient
Karen contacted the Iron Disorders Institute in a panic. She wanted to know why her thirty-year-old husband was severely anemic after a series of phlebotomies, when in fact, his ferritin

had been over 650. It seems her husband had been suffering from chronic fatigue, among other symptoms. Doctors had been baffled, unable to reach a diagnosis. Karen had searched "frantically for answers," as she put it. "The Internet offered the only real hope, and my husband's doctor was ignorant!" she added.

Ironically, the only thing ignorant about her husband's physician was that he allowed himself to be persuaded to perform phlebotomy on this persistent woman's husband, and that he did not order sufficient tests. The husband did indeed have an elevated ferritin, but his transferrin iron saturation percentage had not been checked.

Believing she had the correct and necessary information to get her husband diagnosed and treated, her persistence was intimidating. The physician—probably fearing consequences, such as a lawsuit—did exactly what Karen insisted, which was to begin therapeutic phlebotomy on her husband.

Unfortunately, the man became anemic as a result of phlebotomy; his hemoglobin reached a dangerously low level of 5.0 g/dL before phlebotomies were stopped. It's a small wonder that the woman's husband didn't suffer a heart attack due to seriously low hemoglobin.

What Karen did not learn in her early search for information was that elevated ferritin alone is not enough to warrant phlebotomy. It is, however, a signal to investigate further. In this case, a simple saturation percentage test most likely would have ruled out iron overload as the cause of her husband's symptoms. Elevated ferritin does not always indicate iron loading.

Another Misinformed Patient

Charlene shouted at her pediatrician that her newborn was going to die without a phlebotomy. Hemochromatosis had been diagnosed in her family, and her newborn, whom she had had genetically tested, was a C282Y homozygote. Upon one occasion where she had to make a trip to the family doctor she convinced the doctor to test transferrin iron saturation percentage and serum ferritin on her newborn. When the infant's iron levels came back elevated, the woman panicked. The family doctor admitted he did not know much about hemochromatosis in children and referred the woman to a pediatrician.

When the mother demanded a phlebotomy for her newborn, the pediatrician was both horrified and dumbfounded as to how this woman could have ever reached such a conclusion. The doctor contacted the Iron Disorders Institute to ask for help. He was sent information about pediatric iron levels provided by IDI's Scientific Advisory Board. The information explained that newborns have naturally high iron levels during the first few months of life. Some infants can have a transferrin iron saturation percentage in the high 90 percent range. Infants can also have high serum ferritin levels during this time. Eventually, the pediatrician was able to calm this mother and help her realize that pathologic iron overload in newborns is rare. Among materials sent by IDI was the consideration to test the child at age three for the possibility of an iron loading condition and every five years thereafter until an iron loading pattern might be revealed.

Mothers can become quite agitated, especially when they think their children are at risk for some life-threatening disease. When they hear the term "neonatal hemochromatosis," they don't realize it is a totally different condition from HFE-related hemochromatosis. When they learn that neonatal hemochromatosis is fatal in most cases, mothers can leap to the possibly incorrect conclusion that their newborn's life is in jeopardy. Neonatal hemochromatosis and pathological iron overload in children are discussed in chapter fifteen.

A Physician Who Diagnoses One Case of HHC, Diagnoses an Entire Family
A knowledgeable physician who recognizes that hemochromatosis is common, inherited, and often the cause of multiple symptoms will very likely order the correct tests, provide good therapy, and begin to screen patients who are in high-risk categories.

Names of physicians who are knowledgeable about hemochromatosis is a frequent request made by individuals who contact IDI for information through its Patient Services division. Iron Disorders Institute maintains a database that includes names of physicians who are treating HHC patients. As part of its long-range goals for educating physicians about hemochromatosis, the Iron Disorders Institute encourages each of these individuals to return to their family doctor with literature published by the institute about hemochromatosis. In this way, a physician can learn more about hemochromatosis through his or her patient, while the patient maintains a familiar routine and preserves an already established relationship.

In cases where the person declines to revisit a particular doctor, Iron Disorders Institute Patient Services will provide the individual with a physician's name if available. A package of information about hereditary hemochromatosis is then sent to the person. Another is sent to the former physician.

According to Dr. Vincent Felitti, Director of Kaiser Permanente's Preventive Medicine Department in San Diego where more than 200,000 individuals have been screened for HHC, "Statistically, a family practice physician will likely see one case of homozygous hemochromatosis every two weeks."

Once a physician has successfully diagnosed and treated his or her first case of HHC, it is an eye-opening experience. This physician will become receptive to the possibility of hemochromatosis in anyone who complains of chronic fatigue, joint pain, or any other vague symptoms.

8
Benefits of Screening for Hemochromatosis

Screening for a disease is a technique used to find that disease prior to its causing symptoms or organ damage. Examples of screening include the Pap test, which can detect cervical cancer at a curable stage; the rectal exam for occult blood and prostate enlargement, which can help detect colon or prostate cancer; measuring cholesterol levels to detect possibility of atherosclerosis and potential heart attack; and genetic testing for disorders such as sickle cell trait, Rh-status, and spina bifida. The most common screening test in use is the measurement of blood pressure, an attempt to find and treat high blood pressure before it causes congestive heart failure, stroke, or other blood vessel damage.

Some of these screening measures are automatically used to check a person for disease potential, either at birth with genetic testing, or at given intervals such as pediatric checkups, scheduled visits with the physician such as for college entrance immunization, annual checkups, or work physicals. Other screening can be on a volunteer basis, such as colonoscopy to determine the presence of colorectal cancer, mammography for early detection of breast cancer, and iron panel screening under way at an increasing number of medical facilities.

Including serum iron and key liver enzymes in Executive Panels between years 1990 and 1998 provided a measure of screening for those with hemochromatosis. Elevated serum iron and elevated liver enzymes in both asymptomatic and symptomatic individuals prompted their physician to investigate until the proper diagnosis of hemochromatosis/iron overload was achieved.

Changes in Medicare reimbursement policy resulted in this type of screening mechanism to be removed from Executive Panels. Reinstating serum iron will not happen overnight. Changes in reimbursement policy take months to implement and months to rescind or change. At the IRON2000 USA Scientific Conference of May 2000, hosted by the Iron Disorders Institute (IDI), IDI's Scientific Advisory Board Chairman, Dr. Herbert Bonkovsky, and Vice Chairman, Dr. P. D. Phatak, submitted a letter to the Department of Health and Human Services. This action was in response to Health Care Financing Administration 42 CFR Part 410 Medicare Program negotiated rulemaking proposed changes. These changes were regarding coverage and administrative policies for clinical diagnostic laboratory services and reimbursement of specific tests such as serum ferritin and reflected in proposed rule HCFA-3250-P.

> "SCREENING OF NEWBORNS WITH GENETIC TESTING IS NOT ADVISED. . . ."
>
> —*IRON2000 USA Scientific Conference*

Dr. Bonkovsky and Dr. Phatak's proposed wording provides for reimbursement for cost of serum ferritin for those with elevated fasting transferrin iron saturation percentage.

Screening for Hereditary Hemochromatosis

> "... 45.2 PERCENT OF THE 2,851 PEOPLE PARTICIPATING IN THE CDC SURVEY ABOUT HHC REPORTED THEY WERE DIAGNOSED BECAUSE OF ABNORMAL TESTS PRIOR TO ANY SYMPTOMS OF HHC."
>
> —*U.S. Centers for Disease Control and Prevention 1996 HHC Patient Survey*

What makes routine screening for hemochromatosis, an iron overload disorder, a good idea? Saving lives and money could be compelling enough reasons. Iron overload disorder (disease) meets many of the criteria for population-based screening.

• The disorder is common.

• A sensitive screening test, transferrin iron saturation percentage, exists and allows detection during a long presymptomatic phase.

• A safe, effective treatment is available that can eliminate morbidity (having disease), premature mortality (death), and reduce health costs.

Iron loads in the liver, heart, pancreas, and lungs, as well as in the brain and joints. Iron can interfere with the proper function of most of these organs; moreover, iron is a key nutrient for microbial and cancer cells. Below illustrates the estimated cost to treat a person who has developed iron overload disease. If an iron loading disorder can be detected before accumulation has caused organ damage, the cost to treat could be minor.

DE-IRONING: REQUIRES AN AVERAGE OF 35 UNITS REMOVED OVER AN AVERAGE PERIOD OF 13 MONTHS

MAINTENANCE: REQUIRES 2.1 UNITS REMOVED EVERY 3.2 MONTHS

AVERAGE COST OF SINGLE TREATMENT: $73.07

MEAN AGE AT DIAGNOSIS: 41

—*U.S. Centers for Disease Control and Prevention 1996 HHC Patient Survey*

Hemochromatosis screening and preventive maintenance might include a trip to the family physician, the cost of blood work and a series of phlebotomies, depending on the level of accumulated iron, at an estimated one-time expense of $2,557 per person.

An estimated 1.2 million Americans have hemochromatosis and hence the potential for developing significant iron overload. When diagnosed and treated prior to organ damage, savings are obvious. The maintenance phase of HHC treatment costs

Disease/Disorder	Number Affected	Estimated Annual Treatment Dollars	Yearly Cost Per Person
Cardiovascular	57 million	259 billion	$4,544
Diabetes	16 million	92 billion	$5,750
Cancer	1.2 million	107 billion	$8,917
Liver Disease	25 million	103 billion	$4,120
Arthritis	7 million	15 billion	$2,143

Note: *These costs are used for illustrative purposes and are not all attributable to HHC.*

> "IF THIS HOLDS TRUE, LARGE-BASED POPULATION SCREENING COULD HAVE A SIGNIFICANT IMPACT ON HEALTHCARE COSTS WHEN EARLY DETECTION RESULTS IN TREATMENT. ALMOST NOTHING ELSE WE DO IN MODERN MEDICINE ACTUALLY RESULTS IN COST SAVING THIS WAY."
>
> —*P. D. Phatak, M.D., Head of Hematology and Medical Oncology at Rochester General Hospital, and Vice Chairman, Iron Disorders Institute Scientific Advisory Board*

approximately $600 per year, while treating conditions resulting from iron overload can cost thousands of dollars a year.

The age to begin screening is based on the age when transferrin iron saturation percentage becomes elevated in the majority of individuals with HFE. Mayo Clinic experts recommend that all adults have a transferrin iron saturation percentage test at least once during their lifetime, preferably as a young adult. Iron Disorders Institute recommends family practice physicians consider screening for HHC using transferrin iron saturation percentage by age eighteen, or earlier in high-risk families where an iron loading condition has been established.

Genetic testing as a means of screening for hereditary hemochromatosis is not a practical or cost effective way to identify individuals with this condition. Genetic testing can be expensive, and testing for mutations of HFE currently misses 15 percent of cases of significant iron overload.

Iron overload can occur in children, but when it does, it is usually not HFE-related. This iron overload condition is due to a mutation of other genes such as the one identified by Dr. Clara Camaschella in Italy. She notes that individuals with juvenile HHC (iron overload onset prior to age thirty) do not have known HFE mutations. Instead, they have

> "IT HAS BEEN SUGGESTED THAT GENETIC TESTING COULD BE DONE AT BIRTH AS PART OF NEWBORN SCREENING. GENETIC SCREENING OF NEWBORNS HAS BOTH ETHICAL (LIMITED CONSENT) AND LOGISTIC CONCERNS LONG-TERM FOLLOW-UP."
>
> —*EASL International Consensus Conference on HC Journal of Hepatology 2000*

mutations that occur on the long arm of chromosome 1; the HFE gene resides on the short arm of chromosome 6.

Total iron binding capacity TIBC and UIBC are high in anemias and low in iron overload. UIBC is less expensive than transferrin saturation because it is a one-step biochemical process where transferrin saturation is two steps.

According to an article by iron overload and hemochromatosis expert Dr. Paul Adams, London, Ontario, Canada, "The most established screening test for haemochromatosis is transferrin saturation which is raised in most but not all C282Y homozygotes. . . . The sensitivity of transferrin saturation for the detection of C282Y homozygotes has been reported to be 94 percent in the population screening study from Busselton, Australia, however it was only 52 percent (threshold > 50 percent) in the large study from San Diego."

The U.S. National Institutes of Health HEIRS study on iron overload/hemochromatosis currently underway is incorporating UIBC into the screening process by using it in the calculation of transferrin saturation. Dr. Adams is one of the principal investigators in this study.

9

HFE Mutations Explained

To understand what the terms "homozygote," "heterozygote," and "compound heterozygote" mean with respect to hereditary hemochromatosis, it is useful to keep in mind a few basic facts about human genetics. The genetic material (DNA) comprising a human being is arranged into 46 chromosomes.

One-half or 23 chromosomes, are inherited from each of the parents. Twenty-two of the 23 chromosomes are called the autosomes and the remaining chromosomes, the X- or Y-chromosomes, are called the sex chromosomes because the arrangement of these two chromosomes determines if an individual is a male (XY) or female (XX). Therefore, every human being, with rare exceptions, carries two copies, called homologs, of each of the 22 autosomal chromosomes and either an X and Y, or two X-chromosomes, depending on their sex.

The HFE gene, which when mutated causes hereditary human hemochromatosis (HHC), is located on the short arm of chromosome 6. HHC is considered an autosomal recessive disorder because both copies of the HFE gene, residing on the two homologs of the autosomal chromosome 6, need to have a particular mutation in order for the disorder to present itself. To date, several different mutations in the HFE gene have been described but two in particular, when present in the appropriate arrangement, can lead to the development of HHC.

The major disease-causing mutation is a replacement of the amino acid cysteine with a different amino acid called tyrosine. This mutation is referred to as C282Y. The second disease-causing mutation is a replacement of the amino acid histidine with another amino acid called aspartic acid. This mutation is referred to as H63D. There are additional mutations within the HFE gene, such as S65C and C282S. It is not yet known how significantly these new mutations will contribute to abnormal metabolism of iron. Studies are already under way to determine penetrance of these mutations.

Heterozygote: If an individual has only one mutated chromosome, with any of the HFE mutations, C282Y, H63D, S65C, C282S, etc., the person is referred to as a heterozygote. The remaining nonmutated or good copy of the HFE gene is sufficient in most carriers to prevent the onset of symptoms.

Homozygote: If an individual has the C282Y mutation on both chromosomes, that person is referred to as being a homozygote for the C282Y mutation. These individuals have a very good chance of developing HHC. An individual can also have the H63D mutation on both chromosomes, and this person would also be called homozygous for this mutation. In the United States, approximately 83 percent of all HHC patients are homozygous for the C282Y mutation.

Compound heterozygote: However, if an individual has the C282Y mutation on one of their chromosomes and the H63D mutation on the other chromosome, these individuals can sometimes develop HHC. In fact, of the HHC patients who have the C282Y mutation on only one copy of chromosome 6, approximately 77 percent have H63D on the other chromosome 6. This arrangement is referred to as a compound heterozygote because two different mutations are found together in the same individual.

IRON DISORDERS INSTITUTE GENETICS SERVICES ARE PROVIDED THROUGH GREENWOOD GENETIC CENTER, GREENWOOD, SC.

It was formerly believed that heterozygotes were not at high risk of developing disease, especially if they had one of the lesser mutations of HFE such as H63D or S65C. Since the discovery of C282S, scientists have concluded that this particular mutation is associated with severe iron overload especially when in combination with H63D. Discovery of additional mutations will likely result in an increased number of compound heterozygotes who were formerly classed as heterozygotes.

Examples of HFE Genotypes in Families with Hemochromatosis

x C282Y   • H63D

Both Parents Heterozygous for C282Y Mutation

Children

25% Chance - Normal
50% Chance - Carrier
25% Chance - Homozygous for C282Y

Father Normal (no mutation)   Mother Homozygous for C282Y

Children

100% Chance - Heterozygous for C282Y

If one parent were homozygous for H63D, all children would be heterozygous for H63D.

Father Homozygous for C282Y   Mother Homozygous for H63D

Children

100% Chance - Compound Heterozygous

Father Homozygous for C282Y   Mother Heterozygous for C282Y

Children

50% Chance - Homozygous for C282Y
50% Chance - Heterozygous Carriers

Persons who contact IDI about genetic testing are referred to the Greenwood Genetic Center (GGC). GGC is a nonprofit institute organized to provide clinical genetic services and laboratory testing. They have educational programs and materials about genetics, including genetics counselors. The GGC conducts research in the field of medical genetics. One such study of HFE incidence revealed that C282Y prevalence in the Piedmont region of South Carolina is 1:125 or similar to prevalence in Ireland. Contact information for the center is in the resource section of the book.

10

The Role of a Genetics Counselor

Consulting with a genetics counselor prior to DNA testing is a wise investment in one's health. Genetics counselors are trained professionals with specialized degrees in medical genetics and counseling. They work as members of a team providing information and support to families with a variety of genetic disorders. A genetic counselor can help individuals and families with hemochromatosis In numerous ways, by explaining the pattern of inheritance, identifying at-risk family members, reviewing testing options, and explaining and coordinating genetic testing. These professionals can also point out the benefits and possible consequences of genetic testing as a part of informed consent, which is the legal right of a patient to be informed of the possible consequences of a procedure.

Anyone considering genetic testing should be aware of the consequences. Informed consent can illustrate some of these consequences, such as the fact that once mutations are identified this information is part of your medical history for the rest of your life. Employers and insurance companies can scrutinize individuals with such mutations.

Genetic testing offers invaluable information. Results can provide a long sought-after diagnosis for those with hemochromatosis. Many people with HHC suffer from multiple health problems—none of which completely define the cause of these illnesses.

Gene testing that results in revealing the presence of both mutations of HFE does two things. It provides a solid diagnosis of hereditary hemochromatosis and a great sense of relief and comfort to the patient whose previous diagnoses included hypochondria. Knowing one's HFE status can alert an individual that he or she is in the highest risk category for iron-related disease. If detected early enough, iron-related disease can be prevented. A simple blood donation two or three times a year and modest diet changes might be the only preventive measures these individuals need to observe to avoid potential disease.

The NHGRI is one of the federal agencies in the United States that are charged with taking the leadership on the international effort to map and sequence all human genes, the Human Genome Project. The ELSI Project addresses the ethical, legal, and social implications of genetic testing. The purpose of ELSI is to examine the implications of new developing technologies and information while at the same time studying the basic science, the biology—the actual mapping of the genome.

The intent of ELSI is to assure that genetic technologies are integrated in an appropriate way into clinical and even nonclinical settings and to assure that genetic information will be used appropriately and not used against people to stigmatize or to discriminate.

> "THERE IS NO DOUBT THAT GENETICS WILL REVOLUTIONIZE MEDICINE, BUT CITIZENS NEED TO BE WELL INFORMED ABOUT ANY PROCEDURE THAT HAS LONG-LASTING ETHICAL, LEGAL, AND SOCIAL IMPLICATIONS. NUMEROUS PRIVACY AND DISCRIMINATION ISSUES ARE STILL NOT FULLY ADDRESSED."
>
> —*Elizabeth Thomson, Ph.D., ELSI Program Director, Human Genome Project National Human Genome Research Institute*

The National Institutes of Health National Heart, Lung, and Blood Institute funded a major multi-center, five-year, $30 million clinical trial to actually look at phenotypic and genotypic screening for hereditary hemochromatosis and also for other iron loading conditions. The study involved screening 100,000 people. A study of this magnitude is not without risks; it is possible we may label people who are at the present time healthy. Dr. Thomson points out, ". . . The day will come when if we have enough tests we will all be potentially uninsurable."

11

Who Is a Candidate for Genetic Testing?

Hemochromatosis offers the unique and, possibly, once-in-a-lifetime opportunity to explore and resolve the many issues that accompany genetic testing. HHC is the poster child for this type of testing because HHC is so common; it is treatable, and prevention of disease with early detection can result. HHC can provide the framework for the ethical, legal, and social implications of genetic testing while people benefit from its simplicity as a diagnostic tool.

First, however, questions must be answered and problems resolved about genetic issues, such as privacy. Who will know and who has the right to know about a person's genetic makeup? Who should have access to your information and who should not? What about the legal implications, such as loss of insurance and or employment because of information made knowingly or unknowingly available about a person's genetic condition? These concerns are best illustrated when someone learns that they may have a genetic defect, which could result in an incurable disease such as Lou Gehrig's disease.

Education is key. The Iron Disorders Institute believes that the HFE genetic test is an important and powerful tool. Its application is appropriate when the benefits and risks are fully known and clearly understood from the patient's perspective. Physicians must be sensitive to the proper and improper use of this diagnostic breakthrough and patients must have reliable information about genetics.

Genetic testing can settle issues of whether or not an individual has hemochromatosis. The test confirms the presence of HFE mutation in 85 percent of those who have an iron loading condition. These are remarkable statistics. Genetic testing helps a physician eliminate hours of guesswork, costly lab work, and unnecessary procedures such as liver biopsies. The patient most definitely benefits.

Identifying Carrier Status
Jack Cluster and his two remaining sisters decided to be genetically tested. Two siblings had already died of suspected hemochromatosis; one of liver cancer, the other bleeding esophageal varices, a liver disease–related condition. Their parents had been healthy and had lived well into their eighties. Jack and his two sisters were all found to be C282Y homozygotes. He believes that both his parents were carriers and that all five children inherited both mutations of HFE. Three of those children were confirmed homozygotes; two died of causes commonly associated with undetected hemochromatosis.

Genetic testing of couples who are planning a family to determine carrier status is strongly recommended. An estimated twenty-eight to thirty-two million Americans of European descent are carriers of HFE mutations. This means the children of two carrier parents have a 25 percent chance of getting both mutations and developing health problems.

Females Menstruating or Not
When Jen's grandmother died in 1976, she was told that her death was due to myocardial infarction. Nothing else was ever mentioned; no autopsy was performed. All Jen remembers from that terrible time was thinking, *She's too young to die. She had just turned sixty-nine.*

Over the years Jen had experienced a number of symptoms but not until 1991 would she suspect a connection between these symptoms and her grandmother's death. Jen's severe muscle pain, inability to conceive, heart arrhythmia, chronic fatigue, and even elevated iron levels did not result in the correct diagnosis.

Not until a genetics test revealed she was a compound heterozygote did Jen receive her diagnosis and begin therapy. Had the gene test been available a decade earlier, Jen's story might have a different ending. She is still young enough to have children; she is forty-four, but she and her husband are not certain they will choose parenthood at this late date.

A female's risk for hemochromatosis is the same as a male's. If menstruating, these women have a slightly different loading pattern from males. Monthly blood loss through menstruation provides the benefit of monthly iron loss and therefore a slower rate of iron accumulation.

> "GENETIC TESTING CAN IDENTIFY PATIENTS PRE-SYMPTOMATICALLY; THIS IS ESPECIALLY HELPFUL IN THE CASE OF FEMALES WHO ARE STILL MENSTRUATING."
>
> —*IRON2000 USA Scientific Conference*

When Hemochromatosis Has Been Identified Within the Family
Anyone within the family is at higher risk. Those eighteen or older who have an elevated fasting transferrin iron saturation percentage are good candidates for genetic testing in this situation. Checking iron levels periodically can help a person determine if iron is accumulating, but genetic testing will confirm the diagnosis, eliminate doubt about the presence of the condition, and set a course for therapy, hopefully early enough to avoid disease.

Genetic testing is one of the most powerful new diagnostic tools of the century. Physicians and patients will benefit from the simplicity of the test, but occasionally genetic testing can cause problems. Patients need to be aware of these potential consequences and discuss these fully with their physician.

Informed Consent
Joint pain, chronic fatigue, persistent cough, and heart arrhythmia prompted Tim to see the company physician. Tim's iron levels were elevated, and he was diagnosed with iron overload disease. The company doctor started Tim on phlebotomies through the local hospital system. Tim's boss thought nothing of the periodic blood extractions; he found the notion of too much iron humorous, often making jokes about it. Upon a follow-up exam, the physician casually suggested that Tim get genetically

tested, and Tim agreed. Results showed that Tim was a C282Y homozygote. Thinking this was "interesting news," Tim told his boss that he had a genetic condition called hemochromatosis. Within weeks, Tim was fired, lost his insurance, and had no way to pay for phlebotomy treatment. Had he known the consequences of telling his boss about the genetic outcome, Tim may have never mentioned this to a nonmedical person. Attempts by the physician to enlighten the "boss" about genetics and how Tim would actually have improved health status following phlebotomy failed.

The important thing to keep in mind about genetic testing is that having it done should be a personal and individual decision. Circumstances are different for everyone. There is no reason why a well-informed person should not be genetically tested if there is perceived benefit for that individual.

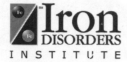**Iron**
DISORDERS
INSTITUTE
PART THREE

Symptoms of Iron Overload

"A COMMON SAYING AMONG PHYSICIANS IS 'SYMPTOMS DON'T HELP DOCTORS RECOGNIZE ZEBRAS WHEN THEY'RE LOOKING FOR HORSES.'"

—*Mark Princell, M.D.,*
Director, Emergency Room Services,
St. Francis Hospital System,
Iron Disorders Institute Scientific
Advisory Board Member

12

Studies, Surveys, and Patient Interviews

"OF THOSE WHO REPORTED SYMPTOMS, 75 PERCENT HAD CHRONIC FATIGUE AND JOINT PAIN."

—*1996 Centers for Disease Control and Prevention HHC Patient Survey*

Jack had been in agony for more than ten years because of severe pain in his hip and finger joints. He was often very tired but thought it was because of stress from the constant pain. Repeated trips to his physician resulted in a prescription for the newest arthritis drug, which offered temporary relief. However, within a few weeks of taking the drug, Jack's liver enzymes became elevated and he had to discontinue the medication.

Having exhausted the list of prescription pain relievers, Jack's physician decided to consult with a colleague who happened to be a gastroenterologist. Measuring Jack's iron levels was suggested. For Jack this triggered a memory of a physical three years earlier, where his serum iron had been elevated. Seemingly unimportant at the time, there was no follow-up to retest serum iron. Now, the significance of this earlier abnormal level is a sobering detail for Jack. An older brother and one sister had just died within a year of one another. His older brother Don had died of bleeding esophageal varices, and his sister Grace had died of liver cancer. "I wonder if they would be alive today?" Jack asks himself. "I also wonder if my arthritic pain would have become so intense. One thing for certain, I would have had fewer phlebotomies," Jack concludes.

Jack's physician, who was not the attending physician three years earlier when abnormal serum iron occurred, ordered a complete iron panel profile, and Jack was properly diagnosed with hemochromatosis. He was able to help two of his sisters, who went immediately to their physician with information Jack had given them about HHC. Both sisters were diagnosed with hemochromatosis. All three were genetically tested and found to be C282Y homozygotes. All received therapeutic phlebotomy and are doing well. Jack's diagnosis was too late to save his brother, who died of bleeding esophageal varices, and his sister, who died of primary liver cancer. He is convinced they had hemochromatosis.

> "LIVER DISEASE SUCH AS CIRRHOSIS AND LIVER CANCER TOP THE LIST OF THE MAIN CAUSES OF DEATH AMONG THOSE WITH HEMOCHROMATOSIS."
>
> —*EASL Consensus Conference on HHC,* Journal of Hepatology *2000*

Many physicians will not make a connection between hemochromatosis and the patient's complaints of joint pain or chronic fatigue. According to a 1996 U.S. Centers for Disease Control and Prevention Survey (see p. 79), chronic fatigue and arthritic pain in joints were the two symptoms most frequently experienced by individuals with hemochromatosis. Chronic fatigue and joint pain were also among the first symptoms to occur in these individuals.

> "EARLY SIGNS OF HEMOCHROMATOSIS ARE WEAKNESS, ARTHRALGIAS, HEPATOMEGALY, AND ELEVATED LIVER ENZYMES."
>
> —*EASL Consensus Conference on HHC,* Journal of Hepatology *2000*

Patient Interviews

The Iron Disorders Institute maintains a database of information about disorders of iron such as hereditary human hemochromatosis, and has done so since early 1997. Information about symptoms, how diagnosis is reached, how individuals become educated about their disorder, and their response to treatment are among data collected.

Prevalence of Selected Signs or Symptoms and Response to Treatment in 2,851 Patients with Hemochromatosis Treated with Phlebotomy

Symptom	Reported Sign or Symptom, Number (%)	Improved with Therapy, Number (%)	Worse Despite Therapy, Number (%)
Extreme fatigue	1,296 (45-5)	705 (54.4)	223 (17.2)
Joint pain	1,241 (43.5)	115 (9.2)	422 (34.0)
Impotence (or loss of libido)	735 (25.8)	93 (12.7)	204 (27.8)
Skin bronzing	733 (25.7)	431 (58.8)	30 (4.1)
Heart fluttering	679 (23.8)	42 (6.2)	69 (10.1)
Depression	592 (20.8)	242 (40.8)	61 (10.3)
Abdominal pain	578 (20.3)	129 (22.3)	69 (11.9)

Frequency of Conditions Reported in the General US Population and US Participants in the Hemochomatosis (HHC) Survey, by Age*

Condition	WOMEN NUMBER (%)		MEN NUMBER (%)	
	General Population	HHC Survey	General Population	HHC Survey
Arthritis				
17-39 years	1,921 (5.9)	10 (10.3)	1,680 (5.2)	15 (8.9)
40-59 years	5,070 (23.4)	147 (34.9)	3,120 (14.7)	194 (22.2)
60-84 years	9,154 (51.1)	212 (42.8)	4,725 (33.8)	203 (31.5)
Diabetes mellitus				
17-39 years	538 (1.6)	3 (3.1)	457 (1.4)	2 (1.2)
40-59 years	950 (4.4)	31 (7.4)	1,087 (1.5)	65 (7.5)
60-84 years	2,437 (13.6)	31 (6.3)	1,991 (12.1)	62 (9.6)
Liver disease or gallbladder disease				
17-39 years	1,887 (7.2)	5 (5.2)	700 (2.7)	16 (9.5)
40-59 Years	2,674 (16.9)	84 (20.0)	1,106 (7.3)	154 (17.7)
60-84 Years	2,135 (25.6)	115 (23.2)	932 (12.2)	113 (17.5)
Extreme fatigue				
17-39 Years	14,235 (43.4)	48 (49.5)	9,647 (29.9)	61 (36.0)

* General population data for liver disease or gallbladder disease from NHANES 11 (1976-1980, reference 19); other general population data from NHANES 111 (1988-1994, reference 20). Arthritis, diabetes, and liver or gallbladder disease based on response to the question: "Have you ever been diagnosed with fatigue by a physician?" Based on self-reported severe fatigue. Data include only white subjects, ages 17 to 84. These data not available in NHANES for older subjects.

Over a period of time, symptoms and signs began to emerge as iron-related. Depending upon which vital organ has been involved, and its function impaired by excessive iron levels, symptoms can be quite varied. Among the most common and typically reported symptoms by individuals with hemochromatosis are:

- joint pain
- chronic fatigue
- loss of libido (sex drive)
- impotence, amenorrhea (premature cessation of menstrual cycle)
- infertility
- sterility
- slow maturation (delayed physical development)
- loss of body hair including baldness
- changes in skin color such as bronzing or reddening, jaundice (yellowish) or ashen gray-olive green-colored skin, redness in the creases of the palms of the hands, dark circles under the eyes
- depression
- elevated cholesterol
- irregular heart beat (arrhythmia) (associated with heart trouble)
- chest pain (associated with heart trouble)
- abdominal pain (associated with liver trouble)
- weight loss (associated with diabetes)
- weight gain (associated with type I diabetes and hypothyroidism)

Other symptoms reported: Symptoms vary from person to person. Sometimes a symptom may seem unrelated until a pattern begins to emerge that seems worthy of consideration. The following list of symptoms were reported to IDI by individuals with hemochromatosis:

- frequent infections
- frequent fever blisters
- rashes
- itching
- blisters on the back side of hands
- fibromyalgia

- irritable bowel syndrome
- excessive thirst and urination
- visual disturbances*
- high blood pressure
- elevated liver enzymes (most strikingly, these were mild)
- elevated hemoglobin/hematocrit
- confusion*
- loss of short-term memory*
- sleep disturbances, including sleep apnea*
- headache (including migraine)
- seizures*
- emotional outbursts*
- moodiness
- attention deficit disorder (ADD)*
- attention deficit hyperactivity (ADHD)*
- restless legs syndrome*
- social withdrawal

Note: All symptoms reported were obtained from individuals diagnosed with hemochromatosis. However, not all these symptoms are common to hemochromatosis. Some of these symptoms * are associated with conditions that can occur in cases of iron deficiency anemia, kidney problems, red blood cell production problems, bone marrow failure, or brain iron maldistribution.

13

Living with Undetected Hemochromatosis

One aspect of hemochromatosis that is not often addressed is the psychological and social impact the disorder can have on a person. Some HHC patients are ashamed to talk about their condition. One newly diagnosed person put it best: "People think hemochromatosis is a blood disease. No matter how I try to explain it, they can't grasp the idea that the only connection hemochromatosis has to blood is that blood is removed to lessen the iron load in the body." Perception, once established, is difficult to change. Hemochromatosis is about excess iron absorption and consequent organ damage, not blood disease.

This misperception about hemochromatosis can only be changed with education, in much the same way people learned about viral hepatitis. Through education, many know that hepatitis A can be contracted easily, hepatitis B and C less frequently than A, and that B and C are more deadly than A. There are preventive measures associated with all three, especially A and B, for which there is a shot or immunization. Through education the same understanding of hemochromatosis can be accomplished. Therefore, as part of the education process, we must include social implications associated with hemochromatosis and its consequences.

Depression
Several individuals with hemochromatosis who have depression claimed that during the time they were trying to obtain diagnosis,

Social Implications
Expressed in Percent Reporting (%)

Type of Change	Severe HHC* (n=1,255)	Without Severe HHC* (n=1,596)
Divorce or breakup with significant other	6.5	2.0
Troubles with spouse or significant other	7.7	14
Marriage or relationship stronger	13.4	4.8
Family members in denial of my disease	12.3	3.8
Family members in denial of own risk	25.2	12.7
Family members supportive	44.5	38.1
Job loss	19.6	2.8
Reduced ability to do daily tasks	33.4	7.3
Loss of health insurance	8.7	5.8
Loss of life insurance	7.7	6.4
Other	5.6	3.3
No real change	28.7	60.0

*HHC- Hemochromatosis

depression was not among the symptoms they provided to their physician. When asked why they had not included depression initially, some said they did not perceive it as related. Others admitted they were too embarrassed to mention it because of the stigma associated with mental illness. Some said that at the time, they did not realize they were depressed until their physician told them so.

Individuals with HHC who contact Iron Disorders Institute often report problems with depression. Whether this depression is situational, or iron related, is not entirely clear. However, if it is iron related, it will resolve with adequate phlebotomy.

Difference Between Fatigue and Depression
Fatigue is when one feels tired and wants to sleep, such as someone who has worked a double shift at the hospital then has to stand up and give a presentation. These individuals are usually interested in life, family, and friends; they are likely happy people, just tired. Their fatigue is readily reversible with rest and is not chronic.

A depressed person has a marked disinterest for life and feelings of sadness. Such persons often are told they seem "blue." A depressed person might remark that they are bored. They may have insomnia or wish to sleep in the daytime to escape contact with people. Change in eating habits and weight can occur with depressed people. Some eat and gain a great deal of weight; some refuse to eat and lose weight. Self-esteem is low and often accompanied by comments of worthlessness and self-doubt. Depressed individuals may have degrees ranging from mild depression to severe. Mildly depressed individuals are able to function but lack motivation. People with severe depression can be suicidal.

> "PRIOR TO 1996, DEPRESSION WAS *NOT* CONSIDERED TO BE A SYMPTOM ASSOCIATED WITH HEMOCHROMATOSIS. OF 2,851 PARTICIPANTS OF THE SURVEY, 344 HAD RECEIVED A DIAGNOSIS OF PSYCHIATRIC DISEASE PRIOR TO BEING DIAGNOSED WITH HEMOCHROMATOSIS."
>
> —*1996 CDC HHC Patient Survey*

A Case of Iron-Related Severe Depression
Craig sat in the front seat of his 1977 Malibu. A .45-caliber pistol lay in his lap. Sheets of rain on the windshield provided a bit of privacy from neighbors who might be passing by. For the past four years Craig's life had steadily gone downhill. He had seen numerous physicians, all of whom eventually came to the same conclusion—that he was a hypochondriac. No matter which doctor he went to, they were never able to find anything remarkably wrong with him, even though he had gained a great deal of weight, was losing his hair, and admitted to impotence and loss of libido. Finally diagnosed with depression, the doctor prescribed Prozac™, which actually made matters worse.

By now Craig had lost his job and his insurance, and friends didn't want to be around him anymore. He felt worthless and couldn't imagine how he could go on even one more day. He picked up the pistol, and cocked it, placing the bullet in the chamber he put the barrel in his mouth and closed his eyes. But he was not able to pull the trigger. Instead, he put the gun back in the glove compartment and wept openly.

Without much thought, he turned the key in the ignition,

starting the Malibu, and headed for his hometown. There he found comfort with his mom and a favorite aunt. Between them they were able to console Craig, assuring him things would improve. He just needed rest and a break from the constant pressure of demands he could not meet. They expressed concern for his depression and encouraged him to move home permanently and to look for another doctor in the area.

It was another year before Craig obtained the proper diagnosis. A persistent, patient, and kind doctor kept searching until a liver biopsy finally provided enough information to confirm the disorder. Craig's liver biopsy revealed 2+ iron and, fortunately for Craig, there was no cirrhosis.

During therapeutic phlebotomy, Craig's depression began to fade. "I don't really remember when it stopped; I just woke up one day and realized I was happy for the first time in six years." Craig says he uses his "mood" factor as a reminder he needs a phlebotomy. He is now a regular blood donor.

Mild Depression

Even though she knew there was work to be done, Martha lacked the desire to get up. Soap operas and game shows served as a distraction and reason not to leave the house except when absolutely necessary. Martha had been to see her doctor about her insomnia, weight gain, lack of energy, feelings of worthlessness, and frequent crying. Several different antidepressants had been prescribed, but the drugs seemed to make her feel worse. Though her fingers, ankles, hips, and knees ached, she did not think these problems were related to her state of mind. She had not always been this way. Martha was practical, hardworking, and active in her church. She loved crafts; she often made decorative picture frames that became gifts treasured by her friends. Now she was ashamed to face those friends because of her inability to "snap out of it," which was the advice given to her by several members of her family.

Martha continued to withdraw from people. Her family doctor told her to seek psychiatric help. She ignored the advice. Two months later at her annual checkup with her gynecologist, Martha was diagnosed with hypothyroidism. She had stopped menstruating at the age of twenty-nine. Her periods had never been regular, and she had given up the idea of having children several years earlier. Though her gynecologist told her that "depression can occur with hypothyroidism," her family members, including her husband, believed that her inability to bear children was the real source of her depression.

On one occasion, when she was trying to "get normal," Martha went to church. She hadn't been in several months and thought it might be good for her. A well-meaning church member draped one arm around Martha's shoulder, squeezing her tightly and shaking her vigorously while offering in a firm, authoritative voice, "You have so much to be grateful for; why not concentrate on all your blessings? Get back to living, young lady!"

A hint of sarcasm could be heard in Martha's voice as she shared this very personal experience. "Most people don't understand depression," says Martha. "It isn't something you choose; it chooses you," she adds. Martha's depression continued for another sixteen months, until she was finally properly diagnosed. A friend of hers had read an article about an iron disorder called hemochromatosis in *Family Circle* magazine and gave it to Martha.

Martha took a copy of the article to her family physician (the one who told her to see a psychiatrist), who initially thought the information was not applicable to Martha. He was concerned that the tests were unnecessary and his patient would experience yet another disappointment. To the doctor's surprise, Martha's serum ferritin and saturation percentage were both elevated.

"I don't blame my doctor," concludes Martha. "He can't possibly know everything. He was visibly shaken when I returned for follow-up after learning my results. I told him to relax; I think he thought I was going to sue him. I was just relieved to know that I was not crazy!" Martha adds and laughs. Martha's mood improved, and her joint pain lessened after ten months of phlebotomies. She is now a regular blood donor.

The cause of depression in people with hemochromatosis/iron overload is not fully understood. Some scientific evidence suggests that the anterior pituitary may be key. Most hemochromatosis experts agree that in the majority of HHC patients who are depressed, this symptom is improved when these individuals are de-ironed and remain so. Other symptoms can be relieved or improved with de-ironing. Some symptoms such as hypothyroidism, infertility, and impotence require medication such as hormone replacement therapy to achieve relief.

Hypothyroidism

Gayle Ryan graduated from nursing school in 1965. She barely remembers the word *hemochromatosis* or the term "bronze diabetes." She became a regular blood donor and learned she was O positive, but it wasn't her blood type that made her curious. While other donors gave blood and left within ten or fifteen minutes, her donation was taking up to forty-five minutes to complete.

In the late 1980s Gayle's younger brother, Thomas, had just returned from a three-month job in the Middle East. Upon return, he had a battery of tests, which included ferritin. Tom's was 4,000, and the physician told him he suspected hemochromatosis. Tom's eyes widened. "That's what my father-in-law died of!" he exclaimed. The physician asked if Tom's wife had ever been checked for hemochromatosis, explaining that it was inherited.

> ". . . THERE IS COMPELLING EVIDENCE FOR CONNECTIONS BETWEEN IRON IMBALANCES IN BRAIN . . . AND HYPOTHYROIDISM, AND LINKS TO HYPOGONADISM AND DEPRESSION ARE STRONGLY SUGGESTIVE."
>
> —*Dr. James Connor, Professor of Anatomy and Neuroscience, Pennsylvania State University, Iron Disorders Institute Scientific Advisory Board Member*

Tom's wife, Jill, had blood work, and they both had a liver biopsy, which confirmed hemochromatosis in Tom and Jill and early cirrhosis in Tom.

Meanwhile, Gayle was still having difficulty with her blood donations, though she continued to go regularly. She was certain that since her brother had been diagnosed with hemochromatosis, she would be too. She knew her "slow-moving, thick blood" was somehow related. But when tested, the doctor told her he saw no signs of the disorder. All he found was a somewhat elevated hemoglobin. Her physician told her to stop smoking and the hemoglobin level would drop.

Three years later symptoms of fatigue, dry itchy skin, hair loss, and weight gain landed Gayle a diagnosis of hypothyroidism, and a prescription for Synthroid. "I pestered the doctor to test my ferritin," comments Gayle. "Finally he gave in; my ferritin was 400." The doctor told Gayle not to be concerned about hemochromatosis; her liver enzymes were normal and she had no symptoms. Gayle insisted that her ferritin be checked periodically. She watched it steadily rise until within a year, her ferritin was up to 800. She asked to be referred to a gastroenterologist. When Gayle heard the gastroenterologist say, "You have no symptoms," she repeated, "I have a ferritin of 800, my brother has hemochromatosis, and my hemoglobin is high; what about a liver biopsy?" The gastroenterologist agreed and performed the biopsy. As Gayle puts it, "much to everyone's surprise but my own, my liver contained 3+ iron!"

After two years of therapeutic phlebotomy under the gastroenterologist's supervision, Gayle changed doctors. She felt the gastroenterologist had lost interest in her. She pointed out that during her two years of therapy under his supervision, he hadn't even palpated her liver. Gayle switched to a hematologist, but as joint disease developed she had to consult with an orthopedist.

Her first twinge of arthritis began in the base of one thumb. Arthritis advanced to the point of needing joint replacement surgery on the entire right hand. Gayle's therapy now includes injections of cortisone into joints in her hands, three times a year. She wears a splint on her hand, writes with "Dr. Grip," and uses "Big Grip" kitchen utensils. She is taking high blood pressure medicine, and often wonders about a paternal aunt who died at age forty-nine of cirrhosis. Most of the family suspected that the aunt might have been a drinker, until they had a personal experience with hemochromatosis. None of Gayle's children have high iron levels; she believes they are carriers.

Impotence
Lucia, a medical technologist, was particularly tenacious in her struggle to discover the cause of the extreme fatigue and pain that sapped her husband Terry's energy. Persistent pain began to insinuate itself into Terry's life during his late teens, particularly in his joints, sides, and legs. He suffered from fatigue and other vague symptoms. But his family doctor could find nothing wrong.

"Doctors just passed the symptoms off as 'I don't know, but you're young and look healthy enough, so it can't be anything major. We'll run a few blood tests,'" Lucia says.

Everyone thought Terry was a hypochondriac and, without a definitive diagnosis as to the cause of his distress, he began to believe he might be. He stopped seeing a doctor and seldom talked about his chronic pain. Eventually his joints hurt nonstop. A rheumatologist performed routine blood work and found Terry's liver enzymes were slightly elevated. However, the doctor dismissed the results and gave him a clean bill of health. Terry was a member of a fraternity at a university and the doctor assumed the elevated levels were due to heavy beer drinking.

> "IMPOTENCE CAN BE CONSIDERED ... A DELAYED SYMPTOM [OF HEMOCHROMATOSIS]; ...UNDERESTIMATING THIS SYMPTOM IS HIGH DUE TO THE FACT THAT, OFTEN, PATIENTS DO NOT SPONTANEOUSLY REPORT THIS SYMPTOM."
>
> —*EASL International Consensus Conference on HC*
> Journal of Hepatology *2000*

As the pain grew worse, another problem arrived. Terry was having trouble getting and holding an erection. He and Lucia did not think the cause was medical. His father had died suddenly at age fifty-five of a pulmonary embolism, and Terry and Lucia were living with his mother to help her deal with his death. Their bedroom was directly above his mother's, so they thought his impotence was due to stress and the awkward location of the bedrooms. But as the year passed, the pain grew worse, the impotency remained, and exhaustion consumed him.

"One night, Terry said to me, 'I'm dying, I feel like I'm dying,'" Lucia says. At the hospital she drew his blood and began checking off every test on the lab order sheet. She had no idea what to look for or what she would find. She did find that his liver enzymes were slightly elevated again. A hospital pathologist suggested he might have hepatitis. After all, Terry was a housekeeper at the hospital, and he was often jabbed by needles when emptying wastebaskets. Although the test for hepatitis came back negative, it provided the first clue to the cause of Terry's constant physical misery. The test showed Terry's iron levels were elevated.

The technician who ran the ferritin test showed it to the laboratory pathologist. The level was so high the instrument couldn't read it. The blood had to be diluted ten times to get a reading. The value was 3,600 ng/mL—normal is up to 300.

"Our laboratory pathologist came to me and said, 'Your husband is very sick,'" Lucia recalls. "The first thing that occurred to both of us was, 'At last, some answers.' Terry wasn't crazy."

The pathologist made an appointment with a liver specialist. Within a week of the appointment, Terry was undergoing a liver biopsy. "The doctor told us Terry would have died had I not run those tests," Lucia says.

Doctors and technicians conducted x-rays and a myriad of tests to discover how much damage had been done to his body. The toll was grim. Terry at age twenty-four had liver damage, arthritis, and nonfunctioning adrenal glands. He was bloated, had blue dots on the insides of his legs from ankle to mid-calf, and dark circles under his eyes. He lacked facial and body hair, and his skin color was gray. But he was alive.

Terry began phlebotomy treatments, but it was two years before his iron levels returned to normal. In the first year after his diagnosis, he was hospitalized four times. He'd often catch colds, leading to bouts with bronchitis and pneumonia.

Today Terry is tall and handsome. His libido is back, and the gray skin color and circles under his eyes are gone. His adrenal functions are normal, and he has a beard and some body hair. Yet he is in constant pain. He still catches frequent colds, which lead to bronchitis. His arthritis is bad, and he continues to have pain in the liver area. Terry now undergoes phlebotomies about once every two months. He absorbs iron so fast that it is difficult to establish a regular maintenance program.

He's prone to episodes of pulmonary embolisms; he's already experienced two. The first destroyed the lower third of his left lung. "I was told I was extremely lucky that I wasn't dead or at the very least a vegetable," Terry says. The second came five years later in the form of multiple blood clots in the right lung. Doctors don't know if the embolisms are related to his iron disorder, and Terry must take the blood-thinning drug Coumadin for the rest of his life.

Lucia works in the blood bank laboratory at the hospital and tries to educate patients about iron disorders, particularly hemochromatosis. She is angered when she hears of cases where iron test results are high but the doctors don't take it seriously. She firmly believes that people need to assume responsibility for researching the cause of their sicknesses if a diagnosis eludes doctors. And they should not be bashful about demanding tests if their symptoms point to a possible cause.

Infertility

"Iron overload disease first showed up in my life in 1971; I was eleven years old," begins Jennifer Hyland, age forty. "Our family physician diagnosed me with viral hepatitis, as my liver counts were off. The hepatitis went away, but my liver counts never reverted to the 'normal' range. My physician at the time even wrote 'hemochromatosis?' in big red letters on my chart. The chart went into his folder, and my physician never thought to follow up on his hunch. My mother never thought to question it either, as the doctor assured us things would be 'just fine.' And somehow, the ball was dropped, and we went back to our normal lives. Meanwhile, I was storing iron every day."

Jennifer's sister Joyce was hospitalized at age forty. After passing out in the street as a result of high blood sugar, she was diagnosed with type 1 diabetes. Although Joyce exhibited many of the same symptoms as Jennifer (arthritis, stomach and headache problems), no one made a connection between the sisters' conditions. Also, not one physician thought to check Joyce's iron.

It wasn't until after Joyce was released from the hospital that a family friend suggested that maybe Joyce and Jennifer had a basic systemic problem. The friend gave Joyce the name of a new physician, and this resulted in Joyce's diagnosis of hemochromatosis, iron overload disease. Joyce was put on a schedule of phlebotomies almost immediately. Jennifer continued her very busy schedule and promising career.

The word *hemochromatosis* was foreign to every member of the Hyland family. They all thought, *Poor Joyce!* Little did they know that this is a hereditary disease. Though Joyce's diagnosis was confirmed, no physician suggested that her siblings be tested. It was at least four months into Joyce's treatment when one of her phlebotomists told her that hemochromatosis was very much an inherited condition. The Hyland family started reading.

By this time Jennifer had moved from New York City to Los Angeles. The move, compounded with losing both a job and a fiancé within weeks of each other, was highly stressful. She was still not menstruating and still had arthritis, which had now been present for three and a half years. Her arthritis had even required surgery on her feet the year before. The surgeons attributed her arthritic feet to an athletic childhood. A connection between her own symptoms and her sister's diagnosis of hemochromatosis had still not been made.

Finally, the research the Hyland family did on HHC/IOD paid off. They realized the necessity of testing each member of the family. "We all got tested immediately, along with our mother, Louise."

Of Louise's five children, two had full-blown hemochromatosis, Joyce and Jennifer. Joyce's ferritin was 2,900. Jennifer's was over 4,900; her saturation percentage was 98 percent.

"Being diagnosed with a disease when you are not feeling 'sick' is a weird thing. It's very easy to just deny it. Yes, I had arthritis and no periods, but I was feeling okay most of the time. I was definitely not prepared for having a 'disease,' especially one that required any kind of treatment! But I took the time to speak to someone more knowledgeable than myself. His name was Dr. William Figueroa. Aside from being one heck of a nice man, he was a respected hematologist at UCLA. He suggested that I get a liver biopsy to confirm the diagnosis. I agreed, as a part of me was still sure that I didn't have this 'disease'!

"Biopsies don't lie," continues Jennifer. "I had hemochromatosis. And to my surprise, apparently so had my father, Tom. He had died at age fifty-eight due to heart and liver failure. He had hemochromatosis all along, and the iron had slowly killed him. Joyce and I had inherited hemochromatosis from our father. But we have learned since the gene discovery that Mom had to be at least a carrier. My sister and I made a vow to him that we wouldn't let it hurt us the way it had hurt him. He had spent years in and out of hospitals with multiple health problems. All the problems we now know to be associated with HHC."

Jennifer, at age twenty-six, began therapy; she endured a long and difficult two years of weakness and problems with anemia and eventually had to give up her job in L.A. and move back home. The last portion of her treatment was the toughest. She endured forced-sustained anemia to ensure that the deep, residual tissue iron was removed. Jennifer felt this was an important part of her therapy.

"I was still not having periods; the doctors had put me on heavy doses of estrogen, in the hopes of 'jump-starting' my reproductive system. The downside to this was that I put on about twenty-five pounds in no time flat! On my worst days, I'd complain that I was not only sick, but I was sick and fat. Mind you, I was 110 pounds at 5'7" before the added weight; not exactly a blimp."

Then a miracle happened. "I woke up one morning, and I was having a period! I never thought I'd be happy to be menstruating, but let me tell you, I was jumping for joy. I was returning to being a normal, healthy functioning human being! It took about a year for my periods to return fully. By this time, I was living back in New York City. I continued to have regular tests on my iron levels as well as my hormonal levels. I had been told by more than one physician that I would not be able to have children, as I was not making any 'follicles,' even following a round of trying out the fertility drug Perganol. This devastated me, but I resigned myself to this being a part of God's greater plan. I was thankful to be healthy for the most part, and decided that I would build the best life I could."

Jennifer's job in New York eventually enabled her to return to Florida when her company relocated to the area. Her new office was within five miles of her mom. Two weeks after arriving back in Florida, Jennifer met a handsome, charming man. They married and several months later, Jennifer experienced what she calls another miracle.

"I woke up feeling very queasy one morning, thinking I had the flu. It lasted for three days until my husband, Wayne, finally came home with a pregnancy test. The test was positive. I told him that was impossible, and he went out and bought four more—each a different brand. Four confirming positive tests meant one thing: I was pregnant! I immediately ran off to the doctor, and she confirmed it. It was the happiest day of my life until the day nine months later, when my son, Adam Jackson, was born.

"Somehow, my life was given back to me in full, and there's not a day that goes by that I am not eternally grateful," recalls Jennifer. "Adam has given me more joy than I could have ever imagined. He is now almost nine years old, and he is as healthy as a horse! He surfs, plays golf, tennis, hockey, skateboards, snowboards, fences, and a bunch of other things. My son has also given me the role of a lifetime—being a mother. And lucky me, I had the best model to learn from—Louise Hyland. Thank you, Mother. Adam and I think of you every day, and we spend our lives living in ways that would make you proud."

Miscarriages, Irritable Bowel Syndrome, and Fibromyalgia
Ellie is a wife, mother, medical technologist, and clinical laboratory science instructor. She would spend twenty-one years trying to get the proper diagnosis of hemochromatosis. Her ordeal began with the first hint of iron overload at age twenty-five when she experienced her first miscarriage. Her second miscarriage took place two years later. Ellie had struggled with infertility, a sign of hemochromatosis, but in time became pregnant after taking Clomid, a fertility drug. Her obstetrician prescribed prenatal vitamins and iron supplements. Soon after starting the iron supplements, she began having intestinal cramps and stopped taking the iron. While pregnant, her hemoglobin remained around 15 g/dL. "My obstetrician remarked that my body seemed to do well being pregnant," remarks Ellie.

"My first actual symptoms appeared when my two children were toddlers. I had recurring bouts of extreme sadness, muscle pain, and fatigue. The fatigue challenged me the most. Considering my lifestyle, it was not surprising that I was tired, even exhausted, on a regular basis. I worked full-time while my husband completed his Ph.D. I pursued my master's degree in Health Sciences in the evenings and continued to care for our two young children."

Then Ellie began having heart palpitations, symptoms of irritable bowel syndrome (IBS), while the aching in her muscles and joints continued. Her family practice physician was the first in a long line of doctors to try to pick at the pieces of her disease. Ellie would see eight different doctors before she was properly diagnosed.

In the early 1990s, one physician noticed slightly elevated liver function tests (LFT) and apparent borderline hypothyroidism. Since elevated LFTs are a sign of possible liver damage, the physician monitored these levels closely. Ellie was told the elevated LFTs were due to a fatty liver.

"The most frightening experience in my search for a diagnosis occurred when a gastroenterologist shocked me with his comment: 'You either have hepatitis, cirrhosis, or liver cancer. I don't think you have hepatitis because you are not sick enough. If you have liver cancer there isn't much we can do for you anyway, and to confirm the cirrhosis, we will have to do a liver biopsy. If we do the liver biopsy there is the danger of hemorrhage.' When I asked him what a liver biopsy would feel like, he replied, 'Like a horse kicked you.' Needless to say, I was not comfortable with Dr. Seven. I agreed, nonetheless, to repeat the blood tests. I did not want to have a liver biopsy—particularly by this physician. Due to my aversion to the biopsy, the doctor ordered a CT scan. I waited, fearful the results would reveal some type of liver cancer. The CT results were normal and an MRI was ordered immediately. I waited again, frightened by the possible results. Nothing was found. Hemochromatosis was never seriously considered in this process. I am not sure it was even mentioned."

The eighth physician was the first to mention hemochromatosis. He explained that this disease was probably more prevalent than we realized and could be treated with phlebotomies. He announced that the only definitive test for this disease was a liver biopsy. Ellie shared her fear of the procedure, and he told her that as long as her iron levels were monitored and she continued to have menstrual periods that the biopsy could be postponed but to be prepared to have the biopsy in the future.

In the summer of 1997, Ellie visited family, which included her cousin, an internal medicine physician. Prior to the visit, Ellie's mother shared with her that this cousin was compiling family information about depression.

"When I questioned him, he clarified that it was not the depression he was researching, but instead the family's liver problems. Our grandfather had died of liver cancer, and my cousin himself had just recently learned that he was a hemochromatosis patient. My husband's response was immediate, 'Isn't that what Dr. Eight thinks you might have?' The referral to the eighth physician had occurred about two to three years prior to this revelation. Suddenly, it clicked! The answers to the puzzle were clear. The elevated LFTs, fatigue, joint pain, heart palpitations, thyroid problems, miscarriages, infertility problems, fibromyalgia, irritable bowel syndrome, and depression were all a part of the same picture. I was certain I had hemochromatosis!"

By this time the genetic testing was available and revealed Ellie was C282Y homozygous for hemochromatosis.

"Looking back on this journey, one key piece of the puzzle that was missing during all those years of assessments was my extended family medical history. If my memory is correct, the medical form that inquired about family medical history asked about parents and grandparents—it did not include aunts, uncles, and cousins. On the paternal side of my family, my father died of pancreatic cancer at age sixty-six. He lived longer than either of his siblings. One of his brothers died of primary liver carcinoma, and the other brother died of a massive heart attack in his late forties or early fifties. My grandparents did not die of illnesses attributed to hemochromatosis, so an abbreviated family history did not pick up the problem that is evident in our extended family.

"People with HHC get frustrated when it is obvious that something must be wrong, but no one can give a justifiable diagnosis. Even when HHC is diagnosed, the correct treatment plan is vague. Guidelines for screening must be determined and extended family histories reviewed. Carriers, as well as those of us homozygous for the disease, need regular monitoring. We want to be confident that the plan for monitoring this lifelong disease is valid. We want all of the medical staff to understand our disease. I am confident our frustrations will lessen, or even disappear, as educational opportunities on hemochromatosis occur. With hemochromatosis, as with other diseases, early detection prevents serious consequences, and means that our quality of life improves dramatically—sooner rather than later," concludes Ellie.

Diabetes, Heart Trouble, and Liver Damage

John straddled the snowmobile. The engine hummed, drowning out noises around him. Bending over, he scooped up a handful of snow, which he promptly ate. His thirst seemed insatiable; no matter how much water he drank, he could not overcome the persistent need for more water. Trips to the bathroom were now a round-the-clock occurrence. As snow melted in his mouth, John was unaware of a fellow snowmobiler barreling toward him from behind. "I vaguely remember the collision," says John. "Mostly I recall being airborne and a terrific pain in one leg, and my gut."

After a painful five-mile-per-hour jostling ride situated on a handmade pine-branch gurney, John was delivered to the emergency room, carried by friends who had seen the accident. Broken bones were of less concern to the emergency room doctor, who suspected internal bleeding. John was rushed to the operating room where the surgeon confirmed a ruptured spleen and noted cirrhosis, as well as a pendulant tumor. "I was conscious when a nurse shouted that my blood glucose was in the 600's, but I passed out at that point," recalls John.

John learned later that he had flatlined. *I'm only forty-one!* John remembers thinking when told the account of his near-death experience. Later in his hospital room, John woke to see his wife, Kay, and his two daughters crying. "I'm fine," John told them, but they cried even harder. John learned later from his wife Kay, a registered nurse and director of hospice, that she had overheard a conversation in the cafeteria that "the McGruder biopsy was likely liver cancer; he's probably a heavy drinker." Kay was shocked at their casualness; she knew John was not a drinker. Kay continued her story, that earlier, while John was on the operating table, one of the surgeons stepped out to ask her how much John drank. "Nothing," she had replied. "He is not a drinker." Kay felt the physician didn't believe her. He explained that John's liver was cirrhotic and a liver biopsy was needed.

The gastroenterologist who had performed the biopsy of

John's liver told his family that he would report the results of the biopsy as soon as they were available. It would likely take two days. "I was a mess," John recalls. "I lay in the hospital room trying to comprehend the events of being revived in the operating room and the possibility that I might have liver cancer. I just kept thinking about my family and what they would do without me."

The gastroenterologist returned two days later with the news; his diagnosis was confirmed as hemochromatosis and diabetes. John's transferrin saturation was 99 percent. He cannot recall his ferritin, or blood glucose level, only that it was seriously elevated.

John remembers, "My mother was a diabetic, and I was told my maternal grandfather and grandmother were as well. Back then, they were never told that there was anything wrong with the iron levels; they probably weren't even tested."

His hemochromatosis was confirmed by second opinion and phlebotomies began. "Two 500 cc units of blood were taken from my body in what was the symbolic precursor to the activity for every day, week, and month from that point forward," provides John. Tests such as saturation percentage and serum ferritin became an important part of John's everyday life.

He jokes about his guardian angel and best friend, Richard, whom he calls Rich. "He killed me and saved my life at the same time." Later Rich would "rat on" John to his physician. During a round of golf, Rich noticed John's shortness of breath and reported it to John's doctor. This resulted in double bypass surgery. "Without his persistence, I might have had a heart attack," adds John.

After sixteen years of faithful compliance with therapy, John still has arthritis, which he describes as the worst part of having HHC. He is still on insulin to control his diabetes, and he watches his diet carefully.

During the course of living with hemochromatosis, John discovered while investigating family history of disease, that a maternal uncle needed phlebotomies for some kind of iron problem. "Because of my experience, I have learned enough about this condition to keep a watchful eye on my family," John shares. "My middle daughter has been diagnosed, thanks to what I have learned. Hopefully, her early detection will keep her

> "SYMPTOMS SUCH AS ABDOMINAL PAIN, WHICH CAN BE ASSOCIATED WITH LIVER DISEASE SUCH AS CIRRHOSIS; FREQUENT URINATION AND UNQUENCHABLE THIRST, WHICH ARE SYMPTOMS OF DIABETES; AND HEART ATTACK, ESPECIALLY AT AN EARLY AGE, ARE AMONG SYMPTOMS [OF HEMOCHROMATOSIS] THAT ARE DELAYED."
>
> —*EASL Consensus Conference on HHC,* Journal of Hepatology *2000*

from unnecessary suffering."

John, now fifty-seven years of age, remarks, "I was raised in Richland, Washington, the Atomic City, and for twenty-plus years, my physical problems were blamed on the 'Down Winder Syndrome' of the Hanford Nuclear site. As much as I have had done, I would like to have something to blame, other than my own body, but being a 'down winder' doesn't amount to the cause of my medical woes, only hemochromatosis can be credited with that."

Symptoms Differ Within Families

Everyone in the Eastman family sat around the Thanksgiving dinner table. Logs crackled in the fireplace, the beautiful fall colors filled the window. Familiar holiday smells of nutmeg and cinnamon floated from the kitchen where pumpkin pie, fresh from the oven, cooled. Norman Rockwell could not have painted a more normal and familiar scene. But things were anything but normal for the Eastmans; they had endured years of seemingly unrelated health problems, without knowing the cause. Everyone in the family had some degree of ill health, but it would be nearly thirty years before Nancy Eastman could put it all together. Now, on this Thanksgiving Day, her family gives thanks to be alive. Even though symptoms varied from person to person within the family, eventually the connection was made.

Nancy was the first person in the Eastman family to be diagnosed with hemochromatosis, followed by the diagnosis of her two sons, two brothers, one nephew, and one sister. She looks across the table at her mother, who was diagnosed thirty-some years earlier with diabetes. Bypass surgery just a few years ago was just the beginning for Nancy's mother. She had terrible sores on her feet that would not heal; and she fell, breaking a leg in the process. Nancy thought about her dad who had died nearly twenty years earlier of a heart attack at age fifty-seven. He had cancer, gallbladder problems, and his autopsy showed an enlarged heart and brown residue in his liver.

She glanced over at her sister, who had suffered with erratic periods, and tried for twelve years before she got pregnant. Eventually she had a hysterectomy. A liver biopsy as a result of Nancy's diagnosis revealed mild cirrhosis and provided the diagnosis of HHC. She was tested genetically and only carried one mutation of HFE, C282Y.

Her older brother experienced his first heart attack at age forty-five and within one year had five bypasses. Now at age fifty-six, he is on full disability. His two sons, Nancy's nephews, have high blood pressure. Her younger brother had been severely depressed for years. When his iron was finally checked his saturation percentage was 62 percent; his ferritin over 300. After phlebotomy treatment he seemed better. His twenty-one-year-old son has a 52 percent saturation percentage; his daughter is anemic. Nancy's youngest brother is thirty-six; he has no symptoms yet, but she is concerned about him.

Nancy thinks back on her own situation. Two difficult births, toxemia, and high blood pressure seemed all just a part of being pregnant. At age forty-four during a routine physical, the physician noted that Nancy's skin looked like that of a person with hemochromatosis. That was the first time she had ever heard the word. No tests were done to see if indeed she had the disorder. Four years later, Nancy returned to her doctor with complaints of abdominal pain, chronic fatigue, joint pain, and depression. This time he mentioned hemochromatosis as a real possibility, tested liver function, and did an iron panel. Liver enzymes were elevated, saturation percentage was 62 percent, ferritin was 1,223. Nancy was referred to a gastroenterologist for a liver biopsy. Hemochromatosis was ruled out. Nancy was given a letter saying so, and she was told to check back with her family doctor in one year, but Nancy did not accept this diagnosis or lack of one.

After some effort, she obtained the original biopsy slides and took her biopsy results letter to another physician, who examined the biopsy slides and diagnosed her immediately. Nancy was glad she had challenged the liver biopsy findings in the letter, especially when the doctor remarked, "I hope we got this before liver cancer." Her therapeutic phlebotomy was begun. After thirteen extractions in twelve weeks, Nancy developed tightness in her jaw and chest. She remembers her doctor saying, "You're too young to be having a heart attack!" A cardiac catheterization revealed an ischemic region (dead tissue) on the inferior (lower) wall of her heart, 50 percent blockage in one artery, and 65 percent in the other. A stent was installed and she was given medication. The pain in her feet, especially toes, kidney infections, red spots on her face, and scalp problems did not seem related to hemochromatosis until, after phlebotomy, these symptoms improved or disappeared entirely.

The Eastman family experience with "unrelated symptoms" spanned nearly ten years. Nancy wonders how different things might be if any one of the four doctors she had seen had been knowledgeable about the symptoms, tests and treatment for hemochromatosis. She misses her dad, but she looks around the Thanksgiving dinner table and gives thanks that the family knows the underlying common denominator of their health problems—hemochromatosis.

Why these symptoms manifest differently among individuals is unknown. Geneticists call this *penetrance*, which means how a gene expresses itself in a person.

A Case of No Symptoms

Fifty-two-year-old Marion had no symptoms of hemochromatosis. She was participating in an HHC screening program at a local hospital in California. At the time Marion was asymptomatic, but she had just gone through menopause. Her ferritin level was 632 with an accompanying saturation level of 71 percent in 1996. Another fifty-two-year-old nurse had a similar experience. She too was participating in a screening program and also was asymptomatic for iron overload. Her saturation percentage was 97 percent and her ferritin was nearly 600 ng/mL. Her liver biopsy revealed a 4+ iron content. For

> "OF 2,851 PARTICIPANTS, 58 PERCENT REPORTED SYMPTOMS, 30 PERCENT HAD NO SYMPTOMS, 12 PERCENT COULD NOT RECALL IF THEY HAD SYMPTOMS."
>
> —*1996 CDC HHC Patient Survey*

the hospital conducting the screening program, hers was one of the highest hepatic iron content levels ever recorded for someone asymptomatic of hemochromatosis.

Some of the symptoms experienced by individuals in these personal stories could have been due to hemochromatosis, but they can also be due to other conditions, such as hepatitis. Also, physicians will see numerous patients who have no symptoms but who actually have hemochromatosis. This helps demonstrate why hemochromatosis cannot be properly diagnosed by symptoms alone and makes a good argument for some type of screening.

14

Body Systems and Excess Iron

Liver
Pain in the upper right quadrant of the abdomen can be a sign of liver damage. Besides the brain, the liver provides more separate functions than any other organ. Situated on the right side of the body beneath the rib cage, the liver weighs $2^1/_2$ to $3^1/_2$ pounds, is 8 to 9 inches in width, and about 6 inches in height. It is concave underneath, covers the stomach, part of the small intestine, gall bladder, right kidney, and right adrenal gland. Among its functions, the liver produces bile, which emulsifies fats; metabolizes carbohydrates, and filters harmful substances such as ammonia, alcohol, drugs, and toxic chemicals. The liver stores cholesterol, vitamins, and clotting factors. It contains macrophages called Kupffer cells, which are scavengers of harmful bacteria and old red blood cells in the bloodstream. The liver also provides for elimination of waste products such as bile pigments, bilirubin, excess cholesterol, lipids, drugs, and poisons.

Everything we eat or drink, including many medications, is processed by the liver. In addition to its metabolic, filtering, defense, storage, and excretion capabilities, our livers have the remarkable ability to function when portions have been cut away. A liver can be surgically resected—the removal of a lobe for the purpose of transplantation—and the remaining portion will not only compensate in function, but will actually generate new cell growth.

Our livers can become diseased in several ways. Viral hepatitis, alcoholism, drugs, exposure to toxic chemicals, excessive consumption of fats, nonalcoholic steatohepatitis (NASH), diabetes, defects in metabolism, and excessively high iron levels as in hereditary hemochromatosis can damage this organ.

There are different types of iron overload; hereditary hemochromatosis is the most common. In the USA, particularly among persons of Northern European extraction, by far the most common cause of hemochromatosis is associated with mutation of the HFE gene. Regardless of the type of hemochromatosis, the liver is the major site for storage of excess iron in the body. Excess iron accumulates in the functional cells of liver; these disproportionately high levels of iron can result in cirrhosis or fibrosis. Any process or organ dependent upon liver function is then compromised.

If a diagnosis of hemochromatosis is made after cirrhosis has developed, the chances that the patient will also develop hepatocellular carcinoma (liver cancer) are increased two hundredfold. At the current rate of detection, approximately 40 percent of patients with hemochromatosis and cirrhosis will eventually develop hepatocellular carcinoma (primary liver cancer). Death is the result for most with this complication unless transplantation with a donor liver can be performed.

The extent of damage to the liver is determined by a liver biopsy. This procedure is currently the only way to absolutely assess liver damage, particularly the presence and degree of scar tissue (cirrhosis, fibrosis).

An excess of iron is toxic to all cells. In large excess, iron alone can cause cirrhosis, liver failure, and hepatocellular carcinoma. In addition to the toxicity of large amounts of iron per se, there is growing evidence that only mildly increased or even normal amounts of iron cause or enhance injury to the liver in the presence of alcohol, fatty liver, chronic viral hepatitis, chronic hepatic porphyria, and probably other hepatotoxic conditions.

Signs of Liver Disease

Other symptoms of liver disease might include nausea, vomiting, jaundice, and ascites (fluid and swelling in the abdominal area). Medical findings such as elevated liver enzymes, serum ferritin levels above 1,000 ng/mL with accompanying elevated transferrin iron saturation percentage, presence of hepatitis B or C, elevated alpha-fetoprotein levels, and abnormal total and direct bilirubin may all be signs of potential or developing liver disease.

One who develops abdominal pain, hepatomegaly (enlargement of the liver), or unexplained weight loss with mild unexplained fever should be evaluated for primary liver cancer.

Cirrhosis

Cirrhosis is the scarring of liver tissue. A leading cause of cirrhosis is alcoholism, but viral hepatitis B or C and hemochromatosis/ iron overload also can result in cirrhosis. Some patients with cirrhosis develop esophageal varices (varicose veins in the lower part of the esophagus). Blood pressure builds in the portal vein, a condition called portal hypertension, causing blood to back up into the esophageal veins. Engorged or bulging veins can rupture due to pressure or be torn by severe coughing, which results in bleeding. These varices can sometimes bleed profusely leading to anemia, and left untreated, a patient can bleed to death.

Portal-Systemic Shunt

A nonsurgical procedure called transjugular intrahepatic portal-systemic shunt, TIPS for short, can be used by patients who are experiencing internal bleeding caused by cirrhosis of the liver. This procedure is also useful for those awaiting liver transplantation. A needle with a balloon catheter is threaded through a vein in the neck into the liver. Except for a moment where it cannot be seen, a contrast dye is used to track the location of the catheter. When the catheter is in the liver, a pathway between blood vessels is created and blood flow through the liver is reestablished. Individuals with portal-systemic shunt are highly susceptible to excessive accumulation of iron.

Hepatitis

More than fifteen years ago scientists began to notice a correlation between elevated iron levels and chronic viral hepatitis. Some speculate iron is released from liver cells injured by the presence of hepatitis virus.

Dr. Baruch S. Blumberg was among the first who noted that patients on dialysis whose serum ferritin levels were lower cleared infection sooner than those with elevated ferritin. Dr. Van Thiel and colleagues were first to observe higher iron levels in association with poor responses to interferon treatment of chronic viral hepatitis. Until recently, interferon was the only treatment available for patients chronically infected with viral hepatitis B or C.

Most patients with hepatitis A, and 95 percent of cases with type B, will realize full recovery and build antibodies against future infection. However, 5 percent of those with type B will remain chronically infected. There is no treatment for type A and approximately one hundred Americans per year die of type A viral hepatitis. There are vaccinations against types A and B. However, with type C, which typically remains with a person for a lifetime, there is no vaccine. Moreover, long-term response to treatment for chronic type C hepatitis is poor; only about 15 to 40 percent improve.

Dr. Van Thiel and colleagues studied seventy-nine patients, all of whom had chronic hepatitis. Serum iron, transferrin iron saturation percentage and ferritin for these patients were measured along with liver biopsy. All the patients were treated with alpha-interferon but only 50 percent responded. Van Thiel noted that liver iron content in patients who did not respond to treatment was twice as high as levels of iron in responders to interferon.

Dr. Herbert Bonkovsky and colleagues Dr. Barbara Banner and Dr. Alan Rothman suggest that patients with viral hepatitis B and C will respond to interferon better when ferritin levels are at about 15 to 20 ng/mL. Further, Dr. Bonkovsky, along with several distinguished scientists including Dr. A. M. DiBisceglie and Dr. Bruce Bacon, studied iron reduction therapy in those with chronic viral hepatitis C. It was noted that liver enzymes alanine aminotransferase (ALT) were significantly reduced in response to interferon treatment when administered following a series of phlebotomies to reduce ferritin.

Assessing Liver Damage

Liver biopsy is used to assess liver damage such as cirrhosis. A small amount of tissue is obtained with a needle and stained with a special iron stain called Perl's stain. Iron will appear blue on the pathologist's slide. Without stain, iron cannot be seen. Another way to identify iron in the liver is with computed tomography (CT scan) or magnetic resonance imaging (MRI) supported with specific laboratory tests.

Formerly, liver biopsy was the most accepted way to diagnose hemochromatosis. Today liver biopsy is used more as a prognostic—the extent to which disease will affect a person—rather than a diagnostic, or the means by which hemochromatosis is diagnosed. For patients who are at high risk for liver cancer, many physicians are screening regularly with serum alpha-fetoprotein (AFP) along with regular hepatic ultrasound or other imaging studies like CT or MRI.

Alpha-fetoprotein (AFP) is a protein used to detect defects in unborn children such as Down syndrome and spina bifida. AFP is also used to detect certain pathological conditions in adults such as tumors. Increased serum AFP levels are found in up to 90 percent of those with hepatomas (liver tumors). Other conditions that can be suspect when AFP levels are elevated include cancers of the lung, stomach, colon, breast, and lymph nodes.

Computerized tomography or CT is produced with x-ray beams that encircle a person. As x-rays pass through the body they are detected by sensors. Information from sensors is computer processed and then displayed as an image on a television-like screen. Sometimes contrast agents are used to block certain tissue from the x-ray. Primary and metastatic tumors will show up as bright white spots on the film.

Magnetic resonance imaging (MRI) uses a large magnet that surrounds a person; radio frequencies interact with the magnet to provide information to the computer. Iron will show up as dark areas on x-rays generated by MRI.

CT scan and MRI procedures do not always reveal mild iron accumulation. They can, however, provide a rough estimate of liver iron content for those who do not wish to have a biopsy performed. Specific techniques must be applied when using CT or MRI diagnostic aids to detect iron in the liver. CT scanning using a dual energy source can detect as little as a two-fold increase in iron stores in a normal liver and a five-fold increase in iron stores in a fatty liver.

Joints

Pain or aching in joints of the hands, especially the first two metacarpal phalanges (knuckles), hips, knees, and ankles are most commonly associated with iron overload. Joint aches or arthralgia is the single most common clinical feature for patients with HHC. Joint pain is very common in the population and hence not specific, but aching of the ankles or of the knuckles and first joint of the second and third fingers (called iron fist) is an unusual pattern that should suggest HHC.

These same hand joints are also often involved in rheumatoid arthritis but in hemochromatosis/iron overload–related arthritis, the patient will usually test negative in the blood for the rheumatoid factor. Rheumatoid arthritis generally attacks a multitude of joints symmetrically and produces a softer, warmer swelling of the joints compared to HHC. Typically a person will have an hour or more of morning stiffness as one of its symptoms. Arthritis in iron overload is commonly misdiagnosed as seronegative rheumatoid arthritis, osteoarthritis, or gout.

SYNOVIAL MEMBRANE

JOINT CAVITY (SYNOVIAL FLUID)

ARTICULAR CARTILAGE

BONE

Any actual arthritis of the ankle, knuckles, or the first joint of the second and third fingers should suggest testing for HHC. The x-ray finding of a white line of chondrocalcinosis in any joint is another tip-off. Chondrocalcinosis or psuedogout is a condi-

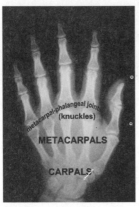

tion of chronic recurrent arthritis clinically similar to gout. In this type of arthritis, patients have calcium pyrophosphate dihydrate (CPPD) crystals but not urate crystals. CPPD crystals can be observed with joint aspiration.

Joint effusions are usually noninflammatory (contain few white blood cells) except when associated with calcium pyrophosphate dihydrate (CPPD) deposition. Dr. Schumacher and his colleagues observed pathologic features of the joint including the cartilage of five patients with hemochromatosis. In addition to the crystal or iron deposits, all had advanced degenerative changes in the cartilage. When iron was seen, it was entirely intracellular (within the cell), where CPPD crystals were commonly seen coating the surface of the eroded cartilage.

JOINT PAIN AFTER INITIAL PHLEBOTOMY	
WORSE	42
SAME	32
BETTER	27
PAIN DURING	15
PAIN AFTER	13

The mechanism by which iron overload causes some patients to develop arthritis remains unknown. A significant number of patients with chondrocalcinosis have underlying hemochromatosis, so it can be a useful marker.

Arthritis was recognized as a manifestation of idiopathic HHC in 1964 by H. Ralph Schumacher. Osteoarthtitis-like changes at the metacarpal-phalangeal (MCP) joints are especially typical of HHC-related arthropathy.

Severe progressive arthropathy can occur despite phlebotomy. Dr. Schumacher, and his colleagues Drs. Pablo Straka, Margaret Krikker, and Andrew Dudley, studied arthropathy in 300 patients with HHC and joint pain. Their findings were based on responses from 159 cases as follows:

EFFECTS OF THERAPY ON JOINT PAIN	HELPED	DID NOT HELP
ASPIRIN	57	6
NSAIDS	32	10
HOT APPLICATION	154	5
COLD APPLICATION	33	109 WORSENED

Treatment

The symptoms of arthritis associated with hemochromatosis can be treated with nonsteroidal anti-inflammatory agents (NSAID), or intra-articular injection of glucocorticoid salts. Other remedies used include:
- Hot compresses and a range of motor exercises
- Oral colchicine
- Oral magnesium carbonate (for possible prevention of CPPD crystals)
- Glucosamine chondroitin for the osteoarthritis
- Ibuprofen (NSAID)
- Phlebotomy therapy

111

Heart

Except for routine blood donors, age fifty-eight is the mean age of death by heart attack in males who die of heart failure due to undiagnosed and untreated hemochromatosis. Family history of heart attack, history of early death by heart failure, or any of the symptoms of impending heart attack listed above—especially heart arrhythmia—are good reasons to ask your physician to examine the possibility that you may have hemochromatosis.

Leading scientists continue to debate iron's involvement in heart disease. Perhaps it would be helpful to distinguish heart disease or cardiomyopathy from coronary artery disease. What is commonly called "heart disease" can either be cardiomyopathy or coronary artery disease. The former is disease of the actual heart muscle; the latter is disease of the artery that nourishes the heart.

Italian scientists Failla, Giannattasio, Piperno, Vergani, Grappiolo, Genetile, and Meles studied radial artery wall alteration in genetic HHC before and after iron depletion. They concluded that in patients with HHC, arterial wall thickness is increased before the onset of cardiovascular complications.

Signs a person may be having a heart attack:

- ☐ pain that radiates up into the jaw and down the left arm
- ☐ irregular heart beat arrhythmia
- ☐ complaints of indigestion or feeling of heaviness in the chest
- ☐ fatigue
- ☐ swelling of feet and ankles
- ☐ shortness of breath
- ☐ ashen-gray color
- ☐ chronic cough
- ☐ sweatiness and anxiety

According to Claus Niederau, M.D., Department of Medicine, St. Josef-Hospital, Academic Teaching Hospital of the University of Essen, Oberhausen, Germany, "For hepatologists, and in particular for physicians and scientists who work in the field of hemochromatosis and iron overload, the data reported by Failla et al., are astonishing and beg the question whether (and if so why) we have overlooked such an association for more than a century."

Niederau continues, "There is overwhelming evidence that cardiomyopathy occurs more frequently in patients with HHC than controls. However, there is also overwhelming evidence that this cardiomyopathy is not caused by coronary artery disease."

A study of records of the U.S. National Center for Health Statistics for years 1979–92 where hemochromatosis was listed as the cause of death provided that "an association of cardiomyopathy (heart disease) and hemochromatosis was increased about 4.8 fold over the expected ratio."

According to the First National Health and Nutrition Examination Epidemiologic Follow-up survey, serum iron levels and transferrin saturation were not related to myocardial infarction. Dr. Chris Sempos et al., even found an inverse association between saturation percentage and coronary heart disease.

Niederau goes on to say, "Recent literature does not support the hypothesis that iron contributes to atherosclerosis to a major degree although further studies are required to elucidate this association. There is overwhelming evidence that atherosclerosis, coronary artery disease, stroke, and peripheral artery disease are neither prominent clinical features nor frequent cause of death in genetic hemochromatosis."

These differences of opinion are not uncommon among scientists. Research is complicated and dynamic. We learn through continued study that new twists and turns of even well-established premises will take place over time. Science adjusts accordingly. As for the heart and hemochromatosis/iron overload, we know that early death by heart attack occurs in hemochromatotics; we may not fully understand the mechanism by which iron contributes to these heart attacks. We can only hypothesize and attempt to prove theory with continued research.

According to the National Institutes of Health, restrictive cardiomyopathy is associated with hemochromatosis/iron overload. Restrictive cardiomyopathy is so named because this condition restricts the heart from stretching properly. While the rhythm and pumping action of the heart may continue to be normal, the stiff walls of the heart chambers keep them from filling normally. So blood flow is reduced, and blood that would normally enter the heart is backed up in the circulatory system. Heart failure is the end result.

Another way iron can contribute to heart failure is through free radical activity, which results in oxidative stress or damage to cells that are involved. Oxidative stress causes cell death and can disrupt the conduction system or electrical impulses within the heart.

Cardiac Conduction System

Arrhythmia is an irregular heart action caused by some disturbance in the discharge of electrical impulses between the sinus node and conductive tissues of the heart. Two separate sounds that help identify murmurs, arrhythmia, or pericardial friction are the "lubb" "dub" sounds associated with the contraction of the ventricle, tension of the atrioventricular valves and the impact of the heart against the chest wall. In a normal heart "lubb" is the first sound heard, followed by a brief pause then the "dub" sound resulting from the closure of the aortic and pulmonary valves. In an arrhythmic heart, pauses are prolonged or erratic.

The heart's conduction system is comprised of a series of electrical impulses or discharges that flow through the heart at a steady and rhythmic pace resulting in a heartbeat. An average heart beats about 72 times per minute. With each beat approximately 80 milliliters (about 1/3 cup) are pumped out of the heart and into circulation. When this system is unable to function normally we have a noticeably irregular heartbeat or arrhythmia.

The conduction system can become impaired in several ways. The functional part of an organ is called the parenchymal (pair-en-ky-mul) cells and it is within these cells that iron can collect. Heavily burdened parenchymal cells can lead to cell death, which can interfere with the flow of cardiac electrical impulses. Another way the conduction system can be impaired is when there is rapid blood loss due to trauma, surgery, or possibly when iron is mobilized too quickly. Mobilization of iron occurs when blood is removed or infused.

Atherosclerosis

Coronary artery disease is the stiffening or narrowing of arteries as a result of specific contributing factors. One well-known factor is a cholesterol-containing component called low-density lipoprotein (LDL). When a particular environment is made available to LDL, plaque may be produced within artery walls. Most scientists would agree that deposition of plaques in the arteries requires oxidation of components such as LDL. Low-density lipoprotein (LDL) is the bad form of cholesterol. LDL has to be oxidized before unique cells called foam cells will trap and process it. The walls of engorged foam cells will gradually enlarge, slowly decreasing the size of the interior of the artery. Diminished blood supply is the outcome of this progression and risk for heart attack is greatly increased. Some scientists speculate that iron, a known oxidant, might be catalyzing the oxidation of LDL and thus contributing to the atherosclerotic process.

When narrowed arteries deprive the heart of oxygen, damage to the heart can occur. Interestingly, the momentary lack of oxygen is not as detrimental as the restoration of the oxygen supply. When blood flow is cut off and thus oxygen deprived, biochemical conditions in the heart are altered. As oxygen reenters the cells free radicals are produced. This causes iron to be released from its storage protein ferritin. Iron amplifies free radical damage, causing potentially irreparable changes to cell membranes and DNA.

People with chronic iron loading disorders such as hemochromatosis and transfusion-dependent iron overload are especially at risk for heart attacks. These individuals must be diligent with iron removal therapy and keep iron levels within a safe range to protect their hearts.

Cardiac diagnostic aids such as electrocardiogram (EKG) will not reveal iron in the heart. A highly skilled cardiologist using an echocardiogram can detect iron. Breakthroughs in magnetic resonance imaging are allowing radiologists to observe iron in the heart with specialized MRI. Using a technique that compares relaxation times between signals, a trained radiologist can produce an image where iron can be seen on an x-ray.

Dr. Herbert Bonkovsky and his colleagues Drs. Richard Rubin, Edward Cable, Ahsley Davidoff, Tammo Pels Rijcken, and David Stark have perfected an MRI method sufficiently sensitive and specific in the estimation of hepatic iron content. According to Dr. David Stark, University of Nebraska Medical Center, this same technique can be applied to imaging the heart.

The presence of iron destroys the signal intensity so that an area with high iron has a low signal and areas without iron have a higher signal. High signals create a pale image; low signals create a black image.

Observing cardiac iron with MRI can provide invaluable information for the physician but this method will not yet disclose how much iron is in the heart. Blood tests such as transferrin iron saturation percentage and serum ferritin are needed to determine the amount of de-ironing that will be necessary to prevent future damage.

> "THERE IS NOTHING THAT CREATES THIS DIFFUSELY BLACK AREA EXCEPT HIGH IRON—PERIOD! IN THE NEW MILLENNIUM IT IS CLEAR THAT MAGNETIC RESONANCE IMAGING, AMONGST ITS MANY CONQUESTS, IS GOING TO CONQUER ANGIOGRAPHY."
>
> —*David Stark, M.D., IRON2000*
> *USA Scientific Conference*

Ferritin, an iron storage protein, traps iron; this mechanism somewhat protects organs against the destructiveness of the metal. Ferritin is contained in nearly every cell of every organ in the human body. The liver produces the greatest amount of ferritin. The heart also produces ferritin but in lesser quantities than other organs—possibly because the heart is a muscle and muscles do not contain large amounts of ferritin.

Among research being conducted in the USA and Canada, scientists at Rammelkamp Research Center in Cleveland, Ohio, are studying how excessive iron affects the hearts of Mongolian gerbils. These furry little creatures seem to have hearts similar in structure to the human heart. Given large doses of iron dextran these gerbils behaved remarkably like humans experiencing iron overload. The animals suffered strokes, arrhythmias, and died prematurely of heart failure similar to humans who have died because of too much iron in tissues such as the heart.

One way in which the gerbils were evaluated was with an electrocardiogram (EKG). Long "Q" wave action was noted in the iron-loaded gerbils. The "Q" wave is the one that follows the "P" wave on an electrocardiogram and is usually not prominent. However, in examples of EKGs of iron-loaded gerbils the extended "Q" wave can easily be seen. Upon autopsy, these scientists were able to determine that in these experimental animals, iron deposits were mostly in the left ventricle and epicardium (outer layer of the wall of the heart). Smaller amounts of iron were present in the right ventricle and atria and within the cells of the heart but not the interstitium (fluid space between heart cells).

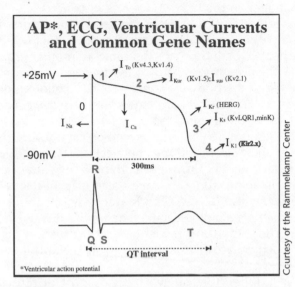

AP*, ECG, Ventricular Currents and Common Gene Names

*Ventricular action potential

Ccurtesy of the Rammelkamp Center

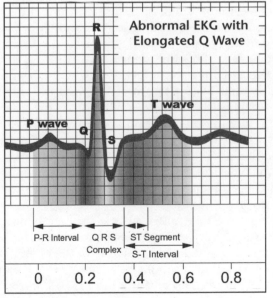

Abnormal EKG with Elongated Q Wave

Brain

Symptoms of depression, seizures, and myalgias are related to iron distribution in the brain.

Iron is stored in the brain in ferritin and transported to the brain and within the brain by transferrin. So the players in the management of brain iron are the same as in other organs. The brain, like the liver, makes its own ferritin and transferrin. Serum ferritin levels in the body are measured in a blood sample taken from the arm. However, brain ferritin levels are determined from fluid obtained from a spinal tap.

Depression is a debilitating psychological disorder that may result from an imbalance in the chemical substances (called neurotransmitters) nerve cells use to communicate with each other. Functional imaging studies have revealed that specific regions in the brain may also be involved in depression, supporting the idea that there is a biological explanation for this psychological disorder. There is strong evidence that depression associated with hemochromatosis may have similar biological underpinnings.

Iron is required for the synthesis of most of the chemical communicators in the brain. Also, those regions in the brain that we know to be involved in motor skills and emotions are also susceptible to iron toxicity. Although the long-established belief in neurology regarding hemochromatosis is that most of the brain is protected against iron overload, the studies upon which this belief is built were performed prior to the technological advances (such as MR imaging for living patients). Additionally enhanced ability to detect iron in autopsy samples is now available. Also, scientists now know there are two issues that are most important about iron in the brain: There must be a balance of iron (can't have too much or too little), and the timing of iron delivery is critical. Even the right amount of iron delivered at the wrong time can be harmful.

The brain has an exquisite system for maintaining a timely balance of iron. All organs have access to iron in the blood, but blood iron is not immediately available to the brain because the blood vessels coursing through the brain are modified to form a barrier between the brain and the blood. This barrier is important for keeping harmful substances in the blood out of the brain. To get required nutrients such as iron and glucose across this barrier, the blood vessels in the brain have carriers. For iron, the blood vessels use transferrin receptors to carry iron in from the blood. These receptors recognize the blood iron transport protein transferrin. Iron in the blood is bound to transferrin. In hemochromatosis (HC), transferrin can be as much as 100 percent saturated with iron, unlike the normal saturation of roughly 30 percent. The high saturation of transferrin in HC may fool the brain into thinking that plenty of iron is available, and the levels of transferrin receptors on the brain blood vessels may decrease to keep too much iron from getting into the brain.

The signals that are used between the brain and its blood vessels to determine how much (and when) iron should be transported into the brain must be discovered before we can directly test this idea. A grant from the National Institutes of Health supported research for scientists James Connor and John Beard to investigate this brain signal function. They proposed that the amount and timely delivery of iron to the brain in hemochromatosis is disrupted as the brain tries to read signals regarding the amount of iron in the blood. Poorly timed or inappropriate amounts of iron delivery to the brain would directly affect the synthesis rates of the chemical communicators for nerve cells, and inappropriate levels of chemical communicators can be associated with depression.

The data supporting the idea that the levels of iron or iron-associated proteins (transferrin or ferritin) in blood can correlate with depression and other psychological illnesses are growing.

Specifically with regard to depression, there is evidence that

> ". . . EXCESS OR INSUFFICIENT IRON IN THE BRAIN CAN CONTRIBUTE TO NEUROLOGICAL DISORDERS. THERE IS A POSSIBILITY THAT THE HEMOCHROMATOTIC BRAIN MAY ACTUALLY BE IRON DEFICIENT. THOUGH PORTIONS OF THE BRAIN ARE CLEARLY CAPABLE OF ACCUMULATING VAST AMOUNTS OF CONCENTRATED IRON, THE BRAIN'S ABILITY TO UTILIZE THIS IRON MIGHT BE IMPAIRED IN THOSE WITH HHC."
>
> —*James Connor, Professor of Anatomy and Neuroscience, Pennsylvania State University and IDI Scientific Advisor IRON2000 USA Scientific Conference*

blood low in iron can be associated with depression in some populations (for example iron-deficient women using the oral contraceptive pill), and depression was a reported side effect in a study using an iron chelator to treat individuals with thalassemia. In the brain, increased iron has been detected with MR imaging in specific regions in depressed patients. A popular therapeutic drug for depression, imipramine, can decrease the ability of a cell to obtain iron. These studies strengthen the argument presented above for a greater understanding of the relationship between iron blood levels and iron brain levels.

Finally, an interesting correlation between depression and activation of the immune systems is developing. The relationship between depression and inflammation may be mediated by a decrease in the amino acid (an amino acid is a protein building block) tryptophan, which is required for synthesis of serotonin. Serotonin is a major chemical communicator in the brain and is the chemical communicator targeted by the popular antidepressant Prozac. The synthesis of serotonin requires iron.

Under conditions of inflammation and immune response, the body tries to minimize iron availability to the invading pathogens by an action referred to as the "iron withholding defense." The leading investigator in this idea is Dr. Eugene Weinberg. In addition, the cells of the immune system use iron to mount their own part of the defense response. Thus, the individual undergoing an immune reaction could get a double whammy of decreased tryptophan and iron withholding from the brain, which combined could have a significant deleterious effect on the ability to make serotonin, which could lead to depression.

In conclusion, the role of iron in the synthesis of chemical communicators in the brain and specifically serotonin is not disputed. The role of serotonin in mediating depression is becoming well established. That hemochromatosis involves a loss of iron balance in the body is the definition of the disorder. Taken together, this information suggests that a specific relationship between iron imbalance and depression would be predicted. Aggressive, targeted studies aimed at understanding the direct link between iron and depression are warranted.

Lower Endocrine System: Pancreas
Symptoms of excessive thirst and frequent and abundant urination, weight loss, and visual disturbances are sometimes related to diabetes mellitus. Hereditary human hemochromatosis (HHC) has diabetes as one of its consequences.

Diabetes mellitus represents a group of disorders that have one common feature: abnormally high levels of glucose (sugar) in the blood. Normally, blood sugar levels are kept within a narrow range (70–130 mg/dL) by several hormonal and neuronal mechanisms, especially by the hormone insulin, which is produced by the beta cells of the pancreas. Beta cells are found in specialized clumps of cells in the pancreas called islet cells. When defects in insulin production, insulin action, or both are present, high blood sugars can result.

Diabetes is usually divided into two broad categories: type 1 diabetes and type 2 diabetes. Type 1 is caused by a deficiency of insulin production by the beta cells in the pancreatic islets, possibly due to viral infections or autoimmune insulitis (inflammation of the beta cells). Type 1 is most common in children and young adults and is often called early onset or juvenile diabetes. Type 2 diabetes is caused by a combination of reduced insulin effectiveness (insulin resistance); there is a concurrent increase in insulin production to compensate for its reduced activity. Individuals with type 2 diabetes initially have too much insulin in the bloodstream or hyperinsulinism. Eventually, however, this type diabetes can result in pancreatic exhaustion and develop into insulin-dependent diabetes. In adults the vast majority of diabetes (about 90 percent) is type 2 diabetes. Because the main cause of type 2 diabetes is obesity, one should be particularly suspicious of hemochromatosis in a thin adult-onset diabetic.

Hypoglycemia—too little blood sugar—can occur in either type 1 or type 2 diabetes. Insulin-dependent diabetics can experience low blood sugars when too much insulin is administered or by failing to eat after insulin has been injected. Type 2 diabetics can experience low blood sugars during the "early" phase when insulin levels are abnormally high if other factors increase glucose utilization or decrease glucose production by the liver.

Although most mild or early diabetics have few or no symptoms whatsoever, symptoms of severe diabetes mellitus may

DIABETES	Type I	Type II
Age at onset	Early (before age 30)	Around age 40+
Symptoms	Frequent & abundant urination Thirst, weight loss Excessive hunger Ketoacidosis: abdominal pain Headache, rapid feeble pulse, Decreased blood pressure, Flushed, dry skin, irritability, Nausea, vomiting, air-hunger/ Shortness of breath, double or Blurred vision	Frequent & abundant urination Thirst, weight change, itching Peripheral neuropathy
Therapy	Insulin & Diet	Diet, hypoglycemic drugs Possible insulin
Islet Cell Antibodies	Present at onset	Absent
Insulin in Blood	Little to none	Present
Body Weight	Normal/under	Obese (80%)
Blood Glucose	Elevated>200mg/dL	Elevated>200mg/dL
Symptoms of HYPOGLYCEMIA	Weakness, Tremor, Muscle twitching, Nausea, Vomiting, Pallor (paleness), Sweating, Confusion, Decreased blood pressure, Decreased heart rate, Palpitations, Air hunger (Shortness of breath, Sighing, Hiccups).	

include frequent and abundant urination, thirst, hunger, weight loss, and blurred vision. The cause of diabetes is not completely understood. Physical inactivity, obesity, and abdominal body fat distribution are all known risk factors for developing diabetes. Presence of diabetes in a family member also increases the risk of development of diabetes, which suggests that genetic factors play a role in causing the disease.

Iron can cause damage to tissues of vital organs by changing oxygen into a form know as a free radical, which leads to increased oxidative stress. Unopposed free radical activity can wreak havoc on cells throughout the body. It may be possible that this is how iron destroys the beta cells, causing diabetes. Beta cells or islet cells have very low levels of the enzymes that break down free radicals. Thus, agents that increase free radical production such as iron could result in destruction of pancreatic cells.

At this time, for those with iron loading disorders such as hemochromatosis, removal of excess iron from the body with therapeutic phlebotomy or periodic blood donation is the safest, cheapest, and most effective way to lower excessive body iron stores. If HHC is diagnosed before complications such as diabetes develop, maintaining a de-ironed status will significantly diminish the risk of iron-related diabetes and other disease for these individuals. Research is under way to determine whether other, more expensive and complicated methods for removing iron will prove to be a benefit in those already with established diabetes-related neuropathy.

"Chelation therapy—inactivation and removal of metals pharmacologically by special chemicals that bind iron tightly— has been shown to slow or even reverse peripheral nerve damage in experimental animals with diabetes," according to Drs. Mingwei Qian of Baylor College of Medicine, Houston, Texas, and John Eaton of the University of Louisville. "It appears that, in diabetes, there is an accumulation of metals such as iron and perhaps copper bound to blood vessel walls. These metal deposits prevent the normal relaxation of blood vessels which feed the nerves and this slowly starves—and ultimately kills—the nerves. This explains why administration of chelators may be able to preserve nerve function even in advanced diabetes, at least in experimental animals."

Chelation therapy for humans with diabetes Is still experimental and calls for additional research such as the study currently in progress in the United States, funded by the National Institutes of Health's Institute for Diabetes, Digestive and Kidney Disease (NIDDK).

Upper Endocrine System: Hypothalamus, Anterior Pituitary, Thyroid
The endocrine system is a highly complex and interdependent network of ductless glands. Glands are organs of the body that manufacture certain substances. The endocrine system discharges its product directly into the bloodstream in the form of hormones, whereas the exocrine glands discharge substances to the outside of an organ to the epithelial tissue. Examples of exocrine system glands include salivary glands, mucous glands, liver, sweat and tear glands, mammary glands, kidneys, stomach, and intestine. It is debatable whether the pancreas is part of the exocrine or endocrine system as it contains both types of glands.

Principal glands that make up the endocrine system include the pituitary, adrenals, pancreas, parathyroid, thyroid, testes, and ovaries. The hypothalamus stimulates pituitary function, which in turn prompts other glands and organs within the endocrine system to produce hormones. Hormones are chemical messengers that regulate specific functions, therefore secretions from endocrine glands are destined for a singular target organ or gland. Properly stimulated target organs and glands provide normal functions such as growth, metabolism, sugar balance, heart rate, breathing, and reproduction.

Sometimes referred to as the master gland, the pituitary produces key hormones. These include thyroid-stimulating hormone, prolactin, oxytocin, luteinizing hormone, and follicle-stimulating hormone, growth hormone, and corticotropin. Two lobes make up the pituitary: an anterior lobe, or front side of the pituitary gland, produces hormones that regulate growth and physical development. This lobe stimulates adrenal function, the thyroid gland, and reproductive organs.

When the pituitary is damaged or function is impaired, hormones cannot deliver their chemical message. Organs relying upon adequate pituitary function are not adequately stimulated and therefore cannot perform their intended function.

Adrenal function: Corticotropin is one hormone produced by the pituitary. It is necessary to the adrenal for making hormones such as cortisone, which acts on fat, carbohydrate, protein, sodium and potassium metabolism, and serves as an anti-inflammatory agent in response to infection or bacteria.

Thyroid function: The thyroid gland produces active substances that affect metabolism and reproductive function. When the thyroid gland is underactive, hypothyroidism is the result. Symptoms of hypothyroidism include chronic fatigue, loss of libido (sex drive), moodiness, low blood pressure, slow pulse, reduced temperature, cool dry skin, brittle nails, hair loss, weight gain, puffy face, dark circles under the eyes, ataxia (lack of coordination), aching muscles, joint stiffness and intolerance to cold, infertility, impotence, sterility, and irregular menstrual periods.

> "ANDROGENS ARE USUALLY EFFICIENT BUT SHOULD BE AVOIDED IN THE CASE OF LIVER DISEASE. . . ."
>
> —EASL International Consensus Conference on HC Journal of Hepatology 2000

The thyroid stimulates other glands to secrete gonadotrophic hormones so that reproduction can take place. Luteinizing hormone (LH) in women causes the release of follicle stimulating hormone (FSH), estrogen and progesterone, and controls reproductive functions such as egg maturation and regulation of menstrual cycle. In males LH causes the release of testosterone and controls the quality of sperm and semen. Gonadotrophins provide for the differences in sexual characteristic of males and females such as voice, body hair distribution, and muscle formation.

Growth hormone (GH) controls the rate of growth of bones and organs and may have some bearing on sleep patterns of males over fifty and postmenopausal females. The pituitary also produces vasopressin, an antidiuretic hormone, which causes the kidneys to retain water, protecting us from dehydration and moderation of blood pressure.

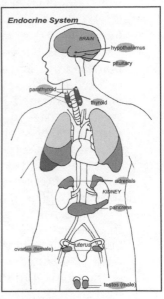

Iron can be detected in the pituitary with MRI (magnetic resonance imaging), but it is not known if iron can safely and completely be removed from this organ. Undiagnosed and untreated iron overload can cause permanent damage to the pituitary gland, resulting in irreversible infertility or impotence.

Testosterone hormone replacement or androgen replacement therapy can be used for cases of impotence. Estrogen replacement therapy can be used for females to stimulate and restore menstruation and ovulation.

Lungs and Iron

We don't typically think of iron as something we inhale; actually, it may seem odd that a heavy metal such as iron can be inhaled. But for fifty years (1925–1975), an even heavier metal, lead, was inhaled in large quantities from automobile exhaust fumes. Indeed, lead is much more hazardous when inhaled than when ingested because the intestinal lining permits only 5–10 percent absorption, whereas the lung allows 30–50 percent entry into the circulatory system.

In the case of inhaled iron, the respiratory tract does have a few defensive strategies. For example, the powerful iron trapping protein, transferrin, is present in lung lining fluid. Further-

125

more, lung defense cells called alveolar macrophages scavenge inhaled iron and deposit it in a protein receptacle termed "ferritin." Gradually, the protein plus the metal is converted into an insoluble precipitate called hemosiderin.

You might ask, how does iron contaminate air and who is at risk of inhaling it? Some sources of airborne iron are obvious—dust from iron mines or smelters or from the grinding or polishing of steel. Other sources are less obvious; these include iron derived from mineral dusts from those types of asbestos that consist of iron silicates, and burning of tobacco. Urban air particulates also are burdened with iron apparently derived from industrial pollution.

Accordingly, we can begin to identify persons at risk. Clearly, workers engaged in ferriferous industries—iron miners, iron smelterers, steel grinders and finishers, asbestos workers, and even nonprofessionals such as persons who scrape tremolite asbestos from surface rocks and use the mineral to whitewash their interior and exterior walls. Not least, we note the extraordinary risk of tobacco smokers as well as the potential risk of persons in the general population who inhale iron from polluted air.

Between 1925 and 1975, numerous studies of iron miners, steel foundry and furnace operators, metal grinders, glazers, and buffers, and steel machinists and turners in Europe and North America reported significantly increased mortality due to cancers of the larynx, bronchial passages, and lungs as compared with workers in non-iron occupations. Not surprisingly, iron workers had markedly elevated ferric oxide contamination in their lungs.

Recent work shows that iron on certain types of asbestos fibers is actually more bioavailable than the iron that is in the crystal structure of asbestos. Asbestos fiber, which once inhaled remains in the lung for a lifetime, will actually acquire iron from the cells in the lung. Lungs can become quite burdened with iron just from the amount of this metal present in one's body. Because these fibers can accumulate iron from the body, it was originally thought that this was a protective mechanism. Thus, it becomes of great significance that these fibers remain in the lung forever after the individual is exposed to the asbestos, and that the iron these individuals accumulate becomes bioavailable and potentially dangerous.

Within the past fifty years, it has become well established that exposure to varieties of asbestos that contain iron silicates can result in malignancies of the lungs and lung lining. The cancers usually appear about twenty or more years after the initial contact with the iron fiber. Varieties of asbestos that consist of magnesium silicates without iron contamination are far less dangerous.

IDI Scientific Advisory Board Member Dr. Ann Aust and her colleagues, experts in inhaled environmental particulates, are examining to what extent bioavailable iron in the urban environment causes acute death. When particle levels in the urban environment rise above a certain level, epidemiologists can predict what percentage of the population will die in the next twenty-four hours from cardiopulmonary problems. Dr. Aust and her team of scientists examined three particular types of coal fly ash: One from Utah, one from Illinois and one from North Dakota. It turns out that these combustion particles are very capable of releasing iron and inducing an inflammatory mediator; the smaller the particle of iron, the more of the inflammatory mediator is released. The smaller the particles, the more damaging to the lung. When iron was removed from the particles using Desferal, a chemical that binds with and removes iron, it completely eliminated the particle's ability to induce this inflammatory mediator.

Iron is carcinogenic in three ways. First, the metal is a powerful oxidant. This action can initiate the cancer process by causing breaks in DNA strands and by changing cellular structure. Second, iron can bolster the growth of cancer cells by suppressing macrophage defenses. Third, iron is an essential nutrient for cancer cell multiplication.

Risk of Infection

As is true for cancer cells, pathogenic microbes likewise grow best in iron loaded tissues. Thus a report recently found that the risk for pneumococcal pneumonia was increased four-fold in current cigarette smokers, and two and one-half fold in passive nonsmokers. Among other infectious diseases markedly increased in smokers are Legionnaires' pneumonia, meningococcal disease, chlamydia pneumonia and Q fever. The latter two infections are especially troubling because these pathogens can, in some patients, be carried by their host macrophages to the coronary arteries to result in cardiovascular damage and death.

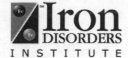

PART FOUR

Hemochromatosis—Not the Only Iron Loading Disorder

"THE FAMILIAR PROTEINS LONG KNOWN TO BE PARTICIPANTS IN IRON SUPPLY AND STORAGE—TRANSFERRIN, TRANSFERRIN RECEPTOR, AND FERRITIN—HAVE RECENTLY BEEN JOINED BY A HOST OF OTHERS. . . ."

—Gary Brittenham, M.D.,
Department of Pediatric Hematology,
Columbia University

15

Other Conditions That Can Cause Iron Overload Disease

Individuals contact Iron Disorders Institute (IDI) on a regular basis wondering if they have hemochromatosis. Some actually do, as confirmed through genetic testing. Some, however, have high iron levels, confirmed with iron panel tests, but they have only one mutation of HFE or none at all. Others have significantly elevated ferritin, but normal transferrin iron saturation percentage.

Hereditary hemochromatosis is not the only condition that results in iron overload. Individuals can have other genetic mutations that cause them to accumulate iron, and they can also have conditions where iron overload occurs because of reasons other than metabolic. For a clear understanding of how hereditary hemochromatosis differs from other iron loading conditions, these disorders are categorized as follows:

Hereditary Hemochromatosis
HFE-related iron overload: These individuals have two mutations of HFE. As a result of both mutations, they can be diagnosed with hereditary hemochromatosis. Therapeutic phlebotomy is warranted for individuals in this category who have elevated ferritin with an accompanying elevated transferrin saturation percentage.

• Homozygote: one who has two of the same of any mutation of HFE (C282Y, H63D, S65C)
• Compound heterozygote: one who has a combination of mutations (C282Y/H63D/S65C)

HFE-influenced iron overload: These individuals have only a single mutation of HFE (C282Y, H63D, or S65C) and express symptoms similar to HHC. They also have elevated saturation percentage, with an accompanying elevated serum ferritin. Therapeutic phlebotomy is warranted for some individuals in this category who have elevated tissue iron without anemia. Others with elevated tissue iron and anemia will require inactivation and removal of metals pharmacologically by special chemicals such as Desferal (deferrioxamine, DFO).

Individuals in this category of iron overload include heterozygotes for any mutation of HFE who have concurrent conditions such as juvenile onset iron overload, African siderosis, hemolytic anemia caused by ineffective erythropoiesis (thalassemia, sideroblastic anemia), other hemolytic anemias, such as G6PD (glucose-6-phosphate dehydrogenase enzyme deficiency), chronic liver disease (viral hepatitis B or C, alcoholic cirrhosis, NASH (nonalcoholic steatohepatitis), primary liver cancer, porphyria cutanea tarda (PCT), aceruloplasminemia, atransferrinemia, neonatal (or perinatal) iron overload, or Friedreich's ataxia.

Non-HFE-Related Iron Overload: These individuals can be the same as those listed in the above category except that these patients have no mutations of HFE. Additionally, the following conditions fall into the category of non-HFE-related iron overload:
- Transfusion-dependent iron overload
- Excessive iron ingestion or parenterally administered iron
- Dysmetabolic iron overload syndrome

Pseudo-iron overload: Individuals in this category may have only one elevated value: an elevated saturation percentage or an elevated ferritin, or an elevated hemoglobin, and no mutations of HFE. Iron overload disease is not highly suspect in this group. Further investigation prior to therapeutic phlebotomy is warranted. Some individuals in this category might benefit from periodic blood donation, but they are not candidates for therapeutic phlebotomy, unless both saturation percentage and serum ferritin are elevated or they have a condition called polycythemia, which is not a disorder of iron but one of overproduction of red blood cells. Pseudo-iron overload can occur in
- Heavy smokers
- Dehydrated persons

- Alcoholics
- Individuals with hepatitis
- Hyperferritinemia-cataract syndrome
- Individuals on hormone replacement therapy
- End-stage renal disease
- Overproduction of red blood cells, such as polycythemia

There is anecdotal evidence at this time that individuals who demonstrate an elevated percentage of saturation with a normal ferritin seem to have as a common denominator sugar imbalances, especially hypoglycemia. Individuals with elevated saturation percentages without elevated ferritin might ask their physician to consider testing HbA_{1c}. This measures blood glucose levels in the preceding five to six weeks. HbA_{1c} should not be confused with Hemoglobin C used to detect certain hemoglobin disorders.

Neonatal and Juvenile Hemochromatosis

Neonatal and juvenile hemochromatosis are rare and not HFE related. Neonates with hemochromatosis usually do not survive longer than two weeks after birth, although there is one documented case of neonatal HC where the youngster not only survived but continued to thrive. The last known report of this child was at two years of age. The origin of neonatal hemochromatosis is unknown.

According to Dr. Clara Camaschella, expert in juvenile hemochromatosis (JHC), the disorder is defined as one who has the appearance of clinical symptoms before the age of thirty. JHC can occur in children or young adults. Dr. Camaschella points out that she and her colleagues have observed only young adults, not children, with JHC, and in each of these cases, their liver function tests were abnormal. She further explains that, when liver biopsy was performed on these patients, liver cirrhosis or advanced fibrosis was always observed in patients twenty years of age and older. She mentions that in a single case, a young patient age fifteen had normal liver function tests, but the liver biopsy showed mild fibrosis. The gene responsible for JHC is on the long arm of chromosome 1 (1q). HFE is on the short arm of chromosome 6.

Transfusion-Dependent or Acquired Iron Overload
Patients with thalassemia major, sickle cell anemia, myelodysplasia (MDS), and some forms of leukemia are often given blood transfusions to correct anemia. Unfortunately, these repeated transfusions can contribute to iron overload. Each unit of blood or single transfusion contains about 250 milligrams (mg) of iron.

Transfusion-dependent patients whose iron accumulation concern is not being addressed are at risk for the same diseases as individuals with hemochromatosis. Thalassemics are especially at risk for heart-related problems. However, widespread organ destruction from excessive tissue iron takes several decades to transpire. When repeated blood transfusion occurs within a relatively short period of time, and excess iron is eventually addressed, organ damage might not be as severe as it can be in persons who have acquired excess iron by other means or who have had elevated tissue iron levels for many years.

Therapeutic phlebotomy is standard treatment for individuals with hemochromatosis, and some cases of acquired iron overload. However, when overload conditions are complicated by the presence of anemia, treatment with an iron-chelating agent such as Desferal™ is the only known way to safely de-iron these patients.

African Siderosis
African siderosis, also called African iron overload, is a common condition in sub-Saharan Africa, where the prevalence of excessive body iron, sufficient to cause organ damage, affects as many as 10 percent of the population in some areas. African siderosis is a condition thought to be associated with a diet high in iron. Some of the iron might be obtained from consumption of a traditional beer drunk by several groups of sub-Saharan Africans. The beer, which is low in alcohol, is brewed in iron drums. Daily consumption of the beer may lead to ingestion of as much as 45 to 85 milligrams of iron per day.

The possibility of a genetic mutation somewhere other than in the HFE gene has been proposed as the cause of African siderosis. According to a 1998 article by Dr. Victor Gordeuk and colleagues, which appeared in the *New England Journal of Medicine*, these scientists measured transferrin iron saturation percentage in 808 African Americans. Their findings showed that 86 percent had normal TS levels, 13 percent had mildly elevated TS levels and 1 percent had highly elevated TS levels, suggesting the presence of as yet undiscovered gene mutations.

Symptoms of African siderosis include elevated sugar, or diabetes, joint pain, heart disease, liver disease, loss of libido, impotence, weakness, fatigue, tuberculosis, malignancies, and osteoporosis due to ascorbic acid deficiency. Africans, or those of African-American descent or black Americans who are homozygous for C282Y mutations of HFE gene, or those who are compound heterozygotes, are also at risk of excess iron accumulation, the same as persons of European descent who have HFE mutations.

Porphyria Cutanea Tarda (PCT)

PCT is a condition of chronic blistering and ulcerating skin lesions, primarily on the dorsal or backs of the hands. Approximately 80 percent of individuals with PCT are infected with viral hepatitis C, and frequently have an HFE mutation. Diagnosis of PCT is usually made by a dermatologist, as some general practitioners might mistake blisters for poison oak or poison ivy. According to Dr. K. E. Anderson of the American Porphyria Foundation, elevated porphyrin levels in plasma and urine are the best indicators of PCT. In some cases, the activity of the defective enzyme uroporphyrinogen decarboxylase is measured in red blood cells. If the activity is decreased in red blood cells, then generally the PCT has been inherited; whereas if red cells are normal, PCT is generally acquired. Treatment for PCT might include discontinuation of alcohol consumption, estrogen replacement therapy, or removal of any offending agent such as toxic chemicals.

Individuals with PCT often require phlebotomy to reduce iron levels and are sometimes given a low dose of chloroquine or hydroxychloroquine, which appears to bind excess porphyrins. Dr. Herbert Bonkovsky, Director, Liver Center and Center for Study of Disorders of Iron and Porphyrin Metabolism, University of Massachusetts Medical School and IDI Scientific Advisory Board Chairman, points out that "retinal damage is a possible side effect of this drug. Patients should have plasma and urine porphyrin levels checked every six months, have regular phlebotomy to reduce iron levels, avoid exposure to sunlight, and should not consume iron pills or alcohol."

Sideroblastic Anemia (SA)
Sideroblastic anemia (SA) is due to an enzyme defect where the body has adequate iron but is unable to incorporate it into hemoglobin. Iron enters the developing red blood cells (erythroblasts); here iron accumulates in the mitochondria—the energy-producing part of a cell—giving a ringed appearance to the nucleus (ringed sideroblast). Red blood cells whose mitochondria are overloaded with iron are unable to form hemoglobin. Sideroblasts are visible with Prussian blue staining and observable under microscopic examination of bone marrow. Because these ringed sideroblasts can develop poorly, or not at all, into mature red cells, anemia is the consequence, while excess iron continues to accumulate in cells. There are two types of sideroblastic anemia: hereditary and acquired idiopathic.

Hereditary SA is due to a genetic defect; the gene is an X-linked (male sex chromosome) recessive (not dominant) gene. It may manifest in both men and women but is seen more commonly in young males, maternal uncles, and cousins. Hereditary sideroblastic anemia generally manifests during the first three decades of life, especially during adolescence, but it has been diagnosed in patients over seventy. Symptoms might include enlarged spleen or liver, liver disease, and cardiac arrhythmia along with specific laboratory findings.

Acquired or acquired idiopathic SA is due to prolonged exposure to toxins like alcohol, lead, drugs, or nutritional imbalances such as deficiency in folic acid, deficiency in copper, or excess zinc. Other causes are due to inflammatory conditions like rheumatoid arthritis, cancerous conditions such as leukemia and lymphoma, kidney disorders causing uremia, endocrine disorders such as hyperthyroidism, and metabolic disorders such as porphyria cutanea tarda. Acquired SA is usually seen in patients over sixty-five years of age, but it can be present as early as mid- to late fifties. Often individuals with this type of sideroblastic anemia develop myelodysplasia syndrome (MDS), which is a bone marrow dysfunctional disorder.

Thalassemia

Thalassemia is an inherited disorder. It is sometimes called Mediterranean anemia, von Jaksch anemia, or Cooley's anemia, after the physician who first diagnosed it.

Genes involved are those that control the production of proteins known as globins, contained in hemoglobin. Hemoglobin production involves two sets of genes on different chromosomes that produce two different pairs of proteins. One set is alpha, the other is beta. Each hemoglobin molecule contains these sets of proteins: two alpha and two beta. Hemoglobin properly binds and releases oxygen when two alpha proteins are connected with two beta proteins. Chromosome 16 controls the alpha, protein set and chromosome 11 controls the beta set. Depending on the genetic outcome from the parents, thalassemia occurs when one or more of the genes fails to produce protein. In alpha thalassemia, one or more of the genes is actually missing. In beta thalassemia, both globin genes are present but fail to produce hemoglobin.

When it is a beta globin gene that fails, beta thalassemia results; when it is the alpha globin that fails, alpha thalassemia results. If one of the beta globin genes fails, the amount of beta globin in the cell is reduced by half. This condition is called thalassemia minor, alpha-thalassemia, or thalassemia minima. If both genes fail, no beta globin protein is produced; this condition is called thalassemia major or beta-thalassemia.

Other forms of thalassemia are minima, intermedia, and E-thalassemia. E-thalassemia is not truly thalassemia; it is considered a hemoglobinopathy (disorders characterized by structural alteration of globin chains), otherwise known as Hemoglobin E, which is not actually thalassemia but rather a mild form of hemolytic anemia. In this disorder, abnormal globins are formed. Thalassemia, on the other hand, is characterized by the inability to produce a sufficient number of globin chains.

People most at risk for thalassemia major, minor, or intermedia are those of Mediterranean (Greek, Italian), Middle Eastern, African, Indian, and Southeastern Asian descent. Hemoglobin E is more common in Southeast Asians, especially in Cambodia, Laos, and Thailand.

With thalassemia major, one can be symptomatic as early as

135

three months of age. In the first year or two of life and in the absence of transfusion, a child can demonstrate severe anemia and expansion of the facial and other bones. These children may be pale or jaundiced, have a poor appetite, fail to grow normally, and have an enlarged spleen, liver, or heart. Because treatment involves frequent blood transfusion (approximately once every month) iron overload will occur. Excess iron accumulates in these organs leading to liver, heart, and pituitary damage and failure of these organs. Other complications of iron overload include diabetes mellitus, hypothyroidism, and hypoparathyroidism. Those with thalassemia intermedia fluctuate between being asymptomatic and having symptoms as severe as those associated with thalassemia major. Diagnosis of thalassemia intermedia is usually made after a period of observation; the decision to transfuse is often a complex one.

Thalassemia minor occurs in heterozygotes who carry the thalassemia trait. These individuals are mostly asymptomatic and have no anemia (except during pregnancy). This trait, however, is being identified in individuals in central and southern Italy who have early onset (before the age of thirty) iron overload, but who do not have the HFE mutation.

Aceruloplasminemia

Aceruloplasminemia is caused by a lack of circulating serum ceruloplasmin, as a result of inherited mutations in the ceruloplasmin gene. Ceruloplasmin, a multi-copper oxidase (enzyme), is required for regulating the efficiency of iron efflux, although the exact mechanism of this is unknown. Individuals who are deficient in serum ceruloplasmin develop both systemic and central nervous system iron overload. Often these individuals are misdiagnosed with hemochromatosis and are phlebotomized. These individuals present with insulin-dependent diabetes mellitus, retinal degeneration, and progressive neuro-degeneration resulting in a Parkinson's-like disease. Ceruloplasmin levels can be measured with a blood test. Laboratory findings in aceruloplasminemia include: absent circulating serum ceruloplasmin (carriers for the disease have one-half the normal levels of ceruloplasmin), mildly lowered serum iron, elevated serum ferritin, and a mild anemia.

Atransferrinemia

Atransferrinemia is a condition in which transferrin, a protein that binds with and transports iron, is absent or deficient (hypotransferrinemia). Severe microcytic, hypochromic (small, pale) red blood cells are detected at birth. Dietary iron is readily absorbed and circulates as unbound iron in plasma. Almost none of this iron can be used to make red blood cells and is instead deposited in the liver, pancreas, kidneys, heart, and thyroid. Little iron is found in the spleen and none in bone marrow. These individuals must receive transferrin by whole red blood transfusions, which can lead to acquired iron overload.

Dysmetabolic Iron Overload Syndrome (DIOS)

DIOS is characterized by elevated ferritin and increased liver iron concentration with normal transferrin-iron saturation percentage. Patients with these characteristics have been described in France and Italy, and it is hypothesized that these individuals represented a subgroup of hemochromatosis.

Friedreich's Ataxia (FA)

Friedreich's ataxia (FA) is caused by a deficiency in the enzyme frataxin. It is a genetic disorder characterized by progressive ataxia, motor weakness, proprioception (loss of awareness of one's relationship to one's body), dysarthria (difficult and defec-

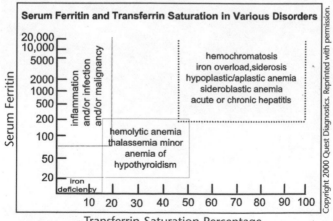

137

tive speech), and cardiac dysfunction. Onset is usually during childhood, with most individuals becoming symptomatic between the ages of eight and fifteen. FA is primarily a disease of the spinal cord and peripheral nerves, but these individuals, for unknown reasons, accumulate iron in the mitochondria (the energy-producing part of a cell) and develop toxic levels of the metal. Frequently an abnormal increase in the size of the heart occurs in patients with Friedreich's ataxia.

These numerous conditions illustrate the complexities and potential dangers of too much iron. When scientists can fully understand the mechanisms by which iron is absorbed, transported, or retained, we will know why these errors in iron metabolism take place. Studies are under way to unlock some of the mysteries about iron and its connection to so many abnormal conditions.

16

Various Roles of Ferritin

"WHEN TISSUE IRON IS SUFFICIENTLY HIGH TO WARRANT ROUTINE PHLEBOTOMY, PATIENTS WILL HAVE NOT ONLY AN ELEVATED SERUM FERRITIN BUT AN ELEVATED TRANSFERRIN SATURATION PERCENTAGE AS WELL."

—IRON2000 USA Patient Conference

Ferritin is an indirect marker of iron and therefore high ferritin levels might represent iron overload. However, not all high ferritin is due to iron overload. Ferritin can be elevated in all, but not limited to the following: hormone replacement therapy, infection caused by bacteria such as E. coli, H. pylori, or yeast such as Candida, viruses such as hepatitis B and C, immune deficiency such as AIDS, inflammation due to alcoholic liver disease, cirrhosis, arthritis, lupus, Crohn's disease, cancer, metabolic disorders such as amyloidosis, and porphyria cutanea tarda, renal disease, and anemia such as pernicious, sideroblastic, hemolytic anemia, sickle cell anemia, and leukemia. Ferritin may also be elevated in other causes of iron overload where no mutations of HFE are present, such as African siderosis, juvenile hemochromatosis, and those who have had repeated blood transfusions or who are transfusion dependent with thalassemia.

Hyperferritinemia—Elevated Ferritin Not Related to Iron Overload Cataract Syndrome
Dr. Donald Brooks, a Professor of ophthalmology, asks, "Are there high levels of ferritin in your blood? Does your doctor think you

may have too much iron in your body? If the answer to either question is yes then you should ask your doctor a further question: Is the serum iron or transferrin saturation also high?"

Several patients with high blood ferritin were referred to hemochromatosis specialists. Unlike hemochromatosis patients, blood tests showed both iron and transferrin saturation to be normal. Liver biopsy also showed normal iron. A breakthrough occurred when it was recognized that the patients with too much ferritin also had cataracts. Examination of family members of each case of persons with high ferritin also had cataracts and conversely those with normal ferritin did not have cataracts. Thus a new disorder called hyperferritinemia cataract syndrome (HCS) was discovered.

Dr. Brooks observes that HCS is a genetic disease that results in excess ferritin production (high ferritin in the blood is called hyperferritinemia) and cataracts. However, unlike ferritin that is high due to iron overload, ferritin is high in HCS with normal or even low iron. Ferritin levels in HCS can range from 500 to 2,500 ng/mL relative to normal levels of less than 220.

HCS was first discovered in 1995 in France and Italy. More than thirty cases of HCS have been diagnosed throughout Western Europe and the United States. At present there is no reason to believe that this disease will be limited to one ethnic group. It is impossible to say how common the disease is because it is simply too new and not enough doctors or patients are aware of HCS. It is possible to miss the diagnosis altogether because HCS patients are generally healthy and may not go to doctors. HCS is typically recognized in patients because of their high blood ferritin.

HCS is also known by the name hereditary hyperferritinemia cataract syndrome to emphasize that it is a heritable genetic disease. It is inherited in a dominant fashion, meaning that an affected parent has a fifty-fifty chance of passing the disease on to each child. Men and women seem to be equally affected. HCS is caused by mutations in a gene that produces the ferritin light chain (L ferritin). All these mutations tend to disrupt a "switch" that normally turns ferritin production off when iron is low. HCS patients make ferritin all the time whether iron is low or high. This ferritin is found in high levels in all parts of the body that have been examined, not just the blood. Genetic testing for mutations that cause HCS is available on a research-only basis.

Cataracts are opaque spots that interfere with passage of light through the normally transparent lens of the eye. People become aware of cataracts when they experience glare, discomfort from bright lights, or are not seeing clearly. Patients with HCS have reported all these symptoms of cataracts. Some people are surprised to learn that they have cataracts as young adults, but usually HCS patients are aware of cataracts before twenty to thirty years of age. The cataracts in HCS have been reported as young as two years of age. The cataracts occur in both eyes and are usually readily apparent to eye care clinicians who put drops in the eyes before a special examination with an instrument called a slit lamp. They appear as numerous, small, dust-like spots.

Currently researchers are trying to discover if there is a connection between ferritin and cataracts. In general, cataracts are the only significant medical problem in HCS patients. Unlike iron overload disorders, there does not appear to be any risk of diabetes or problems in the liver, heart, or joints for one with HCS. A minority of patients with HCS actually have low iron and therefore iron deficiency anemia.

A significant medical problem to be avoided is that of being mistakenly diagnosed as having iron overload. When treated for supposed iron overload by phlebotomy therapy (regular blood donation), HCS patients rapidly develop anemia, fatigue, and breathlessness.

Who should be concerned that they may have HCS? Individuals with blood tests repeatedly showing ferritin above 300 mg/dL with normal serum iron and transferrin saturation should consider HCS. A dilated eye exam by a qualified eye care clinician such as an ophthalmologist would be the next step. If cataracts are found one should discuss this with family members to see if they have high ferritin and cataracts at a young age. If any biological relatives are also found to have both hyperferritinemia and cataracts one should be suspicious that HCS is the cause. A suspected diagnosis of HCS can be confirmed by a medical geneticist, a clinician specially trained in the diagnosis of genetic conditions.

High Ferritin Associated with Defense

Humans have various autoregulated protective systems. One such system that has been discussed frequently throughout chapters in this book is the system that regulates absorption of dietary iron in times of need. Another well-known system is one that protects us when we get an infection. White blood cells race to the site of a wound or to intercept inhaled or ingested microorganisms, which enter the body searching for an opportunity to proliferate and cause disease. Other kinds of white blood cells respond to infection, inflammation, and they clean up debris such as old red blood cells floating in the blood stream. These cells are referred to as macrophages and are present throughout the body.

The scavenging of iron by macrophages is one component of the iron-withholding defense system. Defined by Eugene D. Weinberg, Professor of Microbiology, Indiana University, this simple yet elegant system can be observed to be mobilized in those with chronic malignant, inflammatory, and infectious disease conditions. Individuals with illnesses such as these also will exhibit rising or elevated ferritin.

Whenever dangerous microorganisms, cancer cells, or inflammation is present in the body, the iron-withholding defense system is activated, and more ferritin is produced. Physicians recognize this system but somewhat from a backporch perspective. They know that ferritin increases in the presence of these conditions; for this reason ferritin is called an "acute phase reactant." However, many physicians may not grasp the real reason ferritin reacts during an acute illness. It is a defensive move to protect us from allowing iron to nourish pathogens such as microbial or cancer cells, or to set off free radical activity that destroys cells and DNA.

Several production systems slow down when the iron-withholding defense system is activated. A mild to moderate anemia develops called the anemia of chronic disease. It occurs because the entire body, including red blood cell production, is getting a temporary but modest ration of iron—just enough to get by. Anemia that results in this way may cause some physicians to prescribe iron pills to correct the patient's mild anemia. However, the mild anemia is temporary and will correct itself once the threat of danger is over. Treating the inflammation, infection, or disease present is the best approach. Once the threat of danger is over, systems can return to normal and anemia will fade. Sometimes physicians must ignore this defense system. In advanced cases of disease-related anemia such as cancer, leukemia, and gastrointestinal bleeding, physicians may have to transfuse a patient—even though 250 milligrams of iron are contained in each whole blood cell transfusion. Physicians are properly trained to correct the most acute and life-threatening situation. When patients are in a crisis such as this the decision to transfuse is made in an effort to save a life. Later, once a patient has recovered, therapy can be employed to safely remove the transfusion-obtained iron.

Use of whole blood cell transfusion to address a one-time medical crisis will not necessarily cause iron-related organ damage. Keep in mind, it takes iron several years to accumulate to levels in organs to the extent that irreversible damage is sustained. Meanwhile, when great amounts of iron enter the bloodstream, the human body will step up ferritin production to trap the excess iron.

It should be noted that if a person is seriously iron overloaded prior to transfusion, the system of binding—transport and containment—performed by transferrin and ferritin may be challenged. Under these conditions iron can get loose or free. Unbound by transferrin, iron is like a loose cannon, setting off a chemical reaction called free radical activity. The heart is especially vulnerable during this wild cascade of events caused by iron that is not ushered to its proper place.

Ferritin is safe within a normal range of 25 to 75 ng/mL for those with iron loading disorders such as hemochromatosis. It can rise as high as 200 ng/mL in adult females and 300 ng/mL in adult males without serious health consequences. Elevated ferritin is now being considered a possible indicator of tumor or the presence of cancer, especially pancreatic, colon, lung, breast, testicular, and brain cancers.

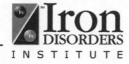

PART FIVE

Battles with Hemochromatosis—
Won or Lost

"Hemochromatosis has claimed the health and lives of too many loved ones. On November 8, 2000, our beautiful daughter, Rhonda, would have celebrated her fortieth birthday. She died March 5, 1984, and was diagnosed at autopsy with hemochromatosis.

"Her death certificate reads 'congestive heart failure due to hemochromatosis.' Rhonda's autopsy report includes hemochromatosis involving heart, liver, cirrhoses, pancreas, spleen, kidneys, adrenal glands, salivary glands, thyroid glands, stomach and duodenum, lymph nodes, and brain.

"Seven years of elevated iron tests provided only one diagnosis: amenorrhea. How was Rhonda's proper diagnosis of hemochromatosis missed?

"Rhonda gave so much in her twenty-three years; but she lives on in a way. As a result of her unnecessary death and this most sobering autopsy report, which cannot be denied, Rhonda will continue to help save many lives. We share this with you in the hope one of those lives might be yours, or that of someone you love as much as we love our Rhonda. She is missed by many."

—*Dolores and Bob Forman*

17

Vital Messages From Two Carriers

The Stories of Charlie Herr & Christopher Main
Medical books lay open on the table of Charlie Herr's hospital room; the pages on hemochromatosis were earmarked. Most of the medical staff had never seen this diagnosis on a chart. Many had never heard of it. Charlie's condition remained critical and then deteriorated. After fourteen days, the decision was made to take him off life support. He passed away peacefully with his family all around him. Hemochromatosis manifested itself in Charlie as arthritis, bronzed skin, and heart disease.

"Dad donated blood regularly. Sometimes he was called in the middle of the night to give when O-negative was in short supply because of an emergency where someone had been in an accident. We realize now that blood donations all those years acted as phlebotomy," notes Laura, one of Mr. Herr's six children. She continues, "Just before Dad's death, we learned from the doctor who diagnosed him, Dr. Michael Novena, that hemochromatosis (HHC) is hereditary. One person in eight can carry a single mutation of the HFE gene, and one in two hundred can carry a double mutation of the HFE gene. We believe Dad had a double mutation. Of the six children, five girls and one boy, some of us were tested immediately, including our mom. She and I tested positive for a single mutation, making us carriers. My brother Chip and sisters Missie, Debbie, Gretchen, and Marcie all were tested. Chip has both mutations, all the rest of us are carriers."

Since Laura was a carrier and knowing that hers sons might be at risk, her husband, Dick, was tested and found to be a carrier as well. Both sons were then tested and found to be homozygotes. Dick and Laura realized at that moment the vastness of HHC. Though they may never manifest symptoms or load iron to excess, their two sons, Chris (age twenty-three) and Matt (age twenty-one), inherited one mutation from each parent, placing them in the highest-risk category for iron overload disease. Chris and Matt both developed symptoms; both loaded iron.

"We learned about hemochromatosis any way we could; our local physicians wanted to help, but they didn't have much information about HHC. The most help came from Dr. Margit Krikker of the Hemochromatosis Foundation, and the Iron Disorders Institute. Dr. Krikker helped us to locate doctors, and IDI supplied us with excellent educational materials about hemochromatosis. Prior to what we received from IDI there were no credible written materials, only photocopied and poorly done folded papers asking for donations.

"Matters were complicated for our sons because they lived out of state, one at college and the other working out west. Chris and Matt had difficulty finding physicians who understood hemochromatosis. One hematologist told Matt, 'Hemochromatosis is an older man's disease and should be of no concern to you now. Watch your diet and alcohol consumption and come back in six months to a year.' At that time, Matt's ferritin was 175 and his transferrin iron saturation percentage was 63. The hematologist made no mention of the need for phlebotomies or further testing.

"Chris's was a different story. He was living in Denver, working at Columbine JDS, a computer software company servicing radio and TV stations throughout the world. Like most of his peers with careers foremost on their minds, health concerns were secondary, especially since Chris felt good. I thought back to when Chris was five. He had been experiencing heart symptoms that baffled his doctors. The odd symptoms followed him into adulthood and were rechecked periodically, but nothing conclusive was determined. Like Dad, who assumed that his arthritis was age-related, the symptoms Chris credited to his being on the go were probably attributable to the insidious HHC damage under way.

"Chris realized the importance of getting treatment and did so. Initially, he required weekly phlebotomy. As his high iron count decreased, the intervals between blood draws stretched to a month with a level check at that time. The goal was to reach and maintain good levels and eventually stretch the treatments to every three months. A new evaluation would determine the frequency of phlebotomies required for the rest of his life."

Chris discovered arranging for phlebotomies proved difficult for a traveler. Often clinics require detailed prescriptions for the draw, and the documentation is not standard everywhere. In some places there is a hefty fee for blood disposal, and in others, the service is free. "Thank you! Red Cross of Columbus, Ohio," interjects Laura. Chris always tried to arrange for his phlebotomy when he was at home.

Every Sunday night Laura and Dick knew that they could count on a call from Chris. This became an established habit and an opportunity for Father, Mother, and son to keep current with each other's lives. Upon learning that Chris was going to begin international travel, Laura reminded her son about updating his immunizations and flu shot and told him that in addition to his hepatitis A, he needed to get the hepatitis B series as well. Laura had learned through both Dr. Sharon McDonnell at the CDC and the Ohio State University travel medicine department that those series were critical.

Shortly before the city of Hong Kong was to be returned to the jurisdiction of the People's Republic of China, Chris accepted his first overseas assignment to Hong Kong. He was thrilled to have such an opportunity and to travel to a place where he could witness first-hand this historic occasion. Sunday evening after a tour on the Mainland, he called home, excited about what he had seen.

But on Monday, Chris began to feel ill. He had been served a questionable meal on the tour. He wondered about contaminated food. His symptoms continued, so he called a doctor but could not get an appointment until Friday. In the meantime he drank lots of fluids (including orange juice from room service) and took ibuprofen for pain relief. He went to work each day. By midweek, the symptoms began to subside and he felt a little better, but he kept the appointment on Friday. When he saw the doctor, Chris didn't think to tell him that he had hemochromatosis. He only told the doctor that he had eaten something he thought might be contaminated and had gastrointestinal symptoms as a result, but by Wednesday he felt better. The doctor prescribed antibiotics and acetaminophen and said if he had any more problems to call back.

That night Chris called home and left a message on the recorder, "Mom, call me. I'm sick. I'll be in my room. Call back any time." Laura was the only one home when she heard the message. She immediately called Chris's room at the hotel. Someone picked up the phone, but there was only silence followed by a dial tone.

"I called back two more times. There was no answer. I called the hotel desk and after considerable pleading, persuaded the night manager to go into Chris's room to check on him. I asked him to call me right back. I waited, all the while knowing something was terribly wrong. The phone call came. The manager, Andy, told me as gently as he could, to sit down and breathe. He then told me that Chris was dead, that the police were in his room, and that I would have to call back on Monday."

Stunned and in disbelief, Laura called her husband. The entire event was surreal, as though they were participants in someone else's tragedy. The next two weeks were somewhat a blur for Dick and Laura Main as they went numbly through the motions of trying to get through each day. Complicated arrangements began with long-distance phone calls until the Mains could get to Hong Kong to claim the body of their son.

When Laura's father, Charlie, died, Laura's husband, Richard, was grief-stricken. He loved Charlie, and spoke of his death as, ". . . a great loss to me, as he was the glue that held the whole group together. He was the one who quietly made things work on a day-to-day basis. He fixed stuff! He loved his grandchildren and all his accumulated sons and daughters-in-law. Even though he was colorblind, he could still sell clothes in a men's clothing department. His loss just left a big hole in my life. I was able to move on, however, knowing that in time we all lose our parents in the natural order of things. Which is why I was dumbfounded, unable to comprehend the death of my son. It is not the natural order of things. It is an event any loving parent fears most but may not vocalize."

Richard shares and continues, "As a dentist, I feel like I have a fairly professional look at diseases and disorders compared to a non-medical person. So, in spite of the fact that complications of hemochromatosis have taken two people from my life, I am still able to look at the disorder in a fairly clinical way.

"Initially, we really didn't have the proper information to have our sons treated adequately; doctors just were not aware. It really makes Laura mad, but I understand that the medical community can't keep up with all the developments in every field. I tried to act strong; after all, I'm the father, husband, man of the family. But soon feelings of disbelief changed to a profound emptiness. I feel as if a part of me has been ripped out and a permanent void remains. I miss Chris every single day. I feel like a vital piece of my future has been stolen. I still find myself waiting for his regular Sunday evening phone call. I don't blame anyone or hemochromatosis for the loss of my son. I just don't think that way. What I do know is that my relationship with my family has suffered. I'm no longer the positive force in their lives. Physically, I'm a mess. Weight gain, lack of exercise, loss of sex drive, and inability to sleep are problems I just can't seem to face and defeat.

"The only thing that I think will heal my open wounds is to stay away from reliving the dreaded events over and over. It just hurts too much to tell and relive the story. I guess I'm looking for distance and time to heal the hurt. I know that my life must go on, and I know that these events can never go away. I want to become me again, but that is impossible. The 'me' I want to be includes being a father to both my sons."

Matt is doing fine at this time. He misses his brother terribly; Chris was his best friend. Matt has many questions about hemochromatosis, and his brother's death is still, for him, unexplained.

Chip Herr, Laura's brother and Chris's uncle, remarks, "When I think of Chris today, how he died, so far from home, I'm filled with overwhelming remorse and anger. If I could just say to people, 'Above all else talk to your family physician about getting tested for HHC. If your doctor looks at you with a blank face, educate him or her! And if the physician is reluctant, force the issue! If that doesn't get results, it's time to look for a new doctor! The test to detect hemochromatosis is just too simple and inexpensive when you consider it might save a life." Chip also has hemochromatosis.

Laura Main is on the Board of Trustees of the Iron Disorders Institute. She speaks to groups every chance she can get to convey the importance of awareness of hemochromatosis. Laura is chairperson for an IDI documentary on hemochromatosis. Her sister, Missie Kendall, an award-winning producer, along with other talented family members, is helping Laura with the film project.

18

Mother, Wife, and Friend

The Story of Irene de Sterke

Irene de Sterke shook her head vigorously, indicating she did not want to have a liver biopsy. Nearly twenty years of being examined, poked, prodded, and cut into without resolve had tarnished her faith in doctors. Liver biopsy seemed just one more unnecessary and invasive procedure. Irene had learned to live with constant chronic fatigue, and pain in her fingers, feet, and knees. After seven major operations to correct ulcerative colitis plus hip replacement surgery, her prolonged illness had left her weary.

Beginning in the mid-1970s, Irene visited her family doctor because of joint pain and incapacitating fatigue. Her husband and children had been concerned about her constant state of tiredness and terrible arthritic pain. When visits to the doctor became a routine event and countless numbers of physicians were unable to get her well, her family began to consider her case hopeless. They wondered if she might be exaggerating her symptoms; maybe this terrible pain she tried to describe was the consequence of something psychological. How could the family possibly know the life of Irene, wife and mother, was in danger? Irene, in fact, was not imagining her pain or fatigue. These symptoms were signals from her body that she was slowly and insidiously being poisoned to death.

Irene de Sterke's health continued to decline. "She became overwhelmed with the pain and fatigue," remembers her son Philip. "Family gatherings were tense. We hated seeing her suffering; it made us feel helpless and cruel for not knowing what was causing her health to be so poor. My sister, Dad, and I tried to comfort her, but we were not the ones experiencing the pain except superficially as bystanders and observers of her agony. We all wanted answers."

Exasperated, Irene finally was referred to a rheumatologist in a major hospital. "This doctor suspected my mother had hemochromatosis," Philip recalls. "But he was not going to treat her without confirmation by liver biopsy." At the time his mother refused to have this biopsy, her ferritin was 6,020 and her saturation percentage was 97 percent. Irene was persistent in her denial of the procedure. Remarkably, her doctor declined to treat her unless she agreed to the biopsy.

Frustrated, scared, and angry, Philip wanted a better understanding of this rare condition called hemochromatosis, and why his mother's doctor felt a liver biopsy was imperative for diagnosis. Enrolled as a student at the University of Amsterdam, Philip had access and knowledge about how to search the library and publications. "I found little information about this 'rare' disease," he remembers. "But from the information I was able to find, I could tell that the biopsy would not be necessary to make the diagnosis and I told this to her doctor. He still refused to treat her without the procedure."

Knowing his mother needed treatment, Philip persuaded her to have the liver biopsy. "I felt like I was taking sides with the doctor against my own mother. She was fearful of the procedure, knowing what it involved. I knew that without the liver biopsy she was not going to get treated. Here in the Dutch Netherlands nearly 99 percent of the population is covered by national insurance. Guidelines are very strict and physicians have to follow them closely to assure the same standard of care for everyone."

Results of Irene's liver biopsy were not surprising to Philip, who by now had read extensively about iron. Her liver was loaded; she had a 4+ iron content. This was exactly what her physician wanted, so that he could confirm his suspicion of hemochromatosis. Therapeutic phlebotomies were started, but because Irene had small veins, the large needles used in standard phlebotomy did not work. In the hospital where she was receiving treatment, some doctors were experimenting with an iron chelator called Deferiprone, also known as DMHP or L1.

Chelators such as deferoxamine (brand name Desferal) can be given intravenously for the purpose of removing iron from patients who have complications such as anemia and iron overload at the same time. Desferal is a chelator that can bind with iron in the bloodstream. Bound iron is then excreted from the body in urine. Deferiprone is a different chelator. It is less efficient than deferoxamine, but it has an advantage in that it can be taken orally.

"As the only alternative to phlebotomy, these doctors decided to give my mother this experimental drug. One and a half years later she died due to hemochromatosis. I could have sued the doctors, but I chose not to. I decided to help educate them instead," Philip continues.

The chelator deferiprone/DMHP/L1 has been approved for use by humans in the European market under the product name of Ferroprox. Several scientists, including Dr. Nancy Olivieri of Toronto's Hospital for Sick Children, have called into question the effectiveness of this drug. During human clinical trials using L1, Dr. Olivieri noted her patients were demonstrating an increased incidence of cirrhosis and that death due to liver failure in patients being given deferiprone was higher than in controls.

"Knowing what I know today, I realize there were a number of choices other than chelation therapy that could have been offered to my mother. She could have had a chest port. A chest port involves the surgical implantation of a device through which blood can be removed or medicines administered. Used primarily by doctors for AIDS and cancer patients, it would have allowed doctors to de-iron her without concern for access to her veins. Mother certainly was a candidate for this procedure because of her extremely high levels of iron and inaccessible veins.

"She also could have had frequent extractions using a small-gauge needle like the butterfly needles used for children and the elderly. Removal of blood twice or even three times a week using this method would have de-ironed her and she might well be alive this minute.

"Also," Philip adds, "she never needed that liver biopsy; I have read about quantitative phlebotomy. Mom could have been diagnosed in this way."

One year after the death of his mother, Philip began to have his own experience with chronic fatigue. "Because of my mother's ordeal, I knew the right tests to ask for," Philip remarks. "My saturation percentage was 60 percentage, but my ferritin was only 250, just slightly increased. I was suspicious that these slightly elevated iron levels could be causing my symptoms, but I too met with skepticism from my doctors. I got tested genetically, thinking this would give me the proof that my iron levels were significant. But as it turns out I am a just a carrier, a C282Y heterozygote.

"Still, my iron levels seemed significant to me. Maybe there were other mutations that contribute to iron loading conditions. I wanted to know if my theory was correct. One thing for certain, regardless of what I might theorize, I knew I was going to have to convince my doctor much the same way I tried to do so for my mom."

Philip began his search for expert proof on the Internet. He remarks, "Not much was available on the subject, and further, what I was able to find was not always correct. I started to contact hemochromatosis patient advocacy groups around the world for advice. I read everything I could find. Some of the best printed material came from the Iron Disorders Institute. However, I wanted to talk face-to-face with an expert, and since I lived half a continent away from the U.S., I continued to look for an expert close to home. Eventually my efforts paid off and led me to a professor, Dr. J. Marx, who specializes in hemochromatosis. Since he lived only twenty miles from me and had an interest in iron loading among HFE heterozygotes. I consulted him. He did some extra tests, and then he agreed with me that some phlebotomies were the best strategy. The results were not major, but I was very happy that the excess iron was removed.

"I didn't know enough about hemochromatosis in time to save my mother, but I was determined to help others before they died like she did," Philip concludes.

Following the death of his mom, Philip de Sterke began an exhaustive and comprehensive search of the Internet and established a website with links to any possible information that might be helpful to people trying to learn about HHC. He went on to found Hemochromatose Vereniging Nederland with a mission to raise awareness among physicians and government agents about hemochromatosis. You can access the Netherlands Hemochromatosis Society website by visiting www.irondisorders.org; go to International links.

Philip closes by saying, "It is a mistake not to take the carrier status seriously. Dr. B. de Valk wrote a very good thesis on C282Y carriers and the risk of heart disease. I recommend everyone read it."

19

Poet, Brother, Husband, and Son

The Story of Sam Martin
Sam Martin was thirty-two when he died unexpectedly on December 31, 1998, from congestive heart failure caused by undiagnosed hemochromatosis.

After a six-day illness characterized by shortness of breath, lack of appetite, fatigue, and low blood pressure, Sam went to his family doctor on December 28. The doctor diagnosed a severe lung and ear infection and sent him home with antibiotics. Early on the morning of Wednesday, December 30, Sam agreed to let his family take him to the hospital.

Emergency room staff at St. Joseph Health Center discovered that Sam had congestive heart failure and an acute diabetic condition. He was transferred to the intensive care unit. Doctors were not sure of the cause of his illness but told family that they thought a massive infection was the most probable. Doctors told Sam's parents and wife late Wednesday morning that he might not survive, and the crisis escalated as more of his vital organs failed. A balloon pump was installed to keep his heart going. He was put on a ventilator and was heavily sedated.

On Thursday, one crisis followed another. Measures that helped one problem worsened others. After Sam's team of doctors discovered that his liver was failing, they began to suspect the hereditary metabolic disorder hemochromatosis. But a definitive diagnosis was not possible at that time; DNA tests would take twenty-four hours and Sam was too unstable for a liver biopsy. After a code blue on Thursday evening he was in a coma. Kidney dialysis worsened his heart failure. Sam died at 11:30 P.M., surrounded by his family. Days later, after a focused autopsy, doctors confirmed that Sam had hereditary hemochromatosis.

Following Sam's death it was found that his father and one sister are carriers of the C282Y gene. His mother is a carrier of both the C282Y and the H63D genes, and his other sister carries the H63D gene. Sam was found to be homozygous for the C282Y mutation.

Hereditary hemochromatosis was not known to be present on either side of Sam's family. On both sides lived relatives who reached advanced age, and there was no history of early death to warn of this genetic time bomb. Sam's death struck his family like a bolt of lightning. When they learned how easily hemochromatosis can be diagnosed and treated, family members were left with much anger at the needlessness of Sam's death.

Sam was the Martins' oldest child and only son. As a boy, he seemed perfectly normal, strong and healthy. He even won physical fitness events in Cub Scouts, and he set a new school record for pull-ups at his elementary school.

Though there were a couple of unusual aspects to his health history, nothing seemed especially serious. At ages three and four, he was evaluated at Children's Mercy Hospital for a heart murmur. After two thorough annual evaluations involving many tests, doctors pronounced his heart normal, just noisy.

Sam had an excellent pediatrician who noted high blood pressure during a football checkup when Sam was fifteen. Again he was referred for evaluation to Children's Mercy Hospital. Several days of testing revealed no obvious problems. Next, an arteriogram was recommended. But since Sam's parents knew him to be a somewhat tense person, they declined that risky procedure and opted for treatment by a doctor who helped Sam reduce his blood pressure through biofeedback training. In later years he took blood pressure medication.

Since Sam's death the Martins have learned that an EKG at that time showed some slight strain or abnormality, though they don't remember hearing about it then. They wonder, could that arteriogram have revealed his hemochromatosis?

Sam's physical health as a young man seemed okay. Although he took blood pressure medication and an antidepressant, he seemed to have normal physical health and energy.

Sam had several symptoms of hemochromatosis in his last year or two, but they were easy to attribute to other causes. The pain in his neck and back seemed to result from a rear-end auto accident, and his fatigue seemed related to his repeated attempts to give up smokeless tobacco. Sam was more likely to visit the health food store seeking ways to help himself than to visit his doctor. He used herbs such as gingko biloba and ginseng. He underwent Rolfing treatments.

Sam's doctor for his last five years, an osteopathic physician, never ordered iron tests. Routine screening and diagnosis when he was much younger would have saved Sam's life and health.

Sam is survived by his parents, James and Sidney Martin; his wife, Lucinda Martin; and his sisters, Rachel and Hannah Martin.

Sam was a poet, photographer, gardener, stained glass artist, bird lover, connoisseur of Mexican food, and an aspiring guitarist. He was a lifelong Kansas City resident and worked at a print shop. His family remembers him most as a loving brother and son, and the most kind and spiritual person they have known. Without him, the Martin family will never be the same.

The Martins are grateful to the St. Joseph Health Center doctors and staff, who worked heroically for forty-two hours on Sam's behalf and who treated them with compassion. But questions still plague them. Why did Sam die so young from hemochromatosis? Did he have a heart defect that contributed to his death? Did he accumulate iron faster through his diet or use of tobacco? Did other genetic factors hasten the development of the disorder? If hemochromatosis usually kills at age fifty or sixty, why did Sam die at thirty-two?

Sam's final diagnosis included:
1. End-stage dilated cardiomyopathy with congestive heart failure
2. Liver failure
3. Renal failure
4. Upper gastrointestinal bleeding
5. Disseminated intravascular coagulation
6. Hemochromatosis

Sam's autopsy states that he died from multisystem failure due to hemochromatosis.

The report mentions a history of hypertension. Noted on the anatomic portion of the report is cardiac failure, hepatic cirrhosis, pancreatic insufficiency, renal insufficiency, coagulapathy, gastric hemorrhage, bilateral pleural effusions, and ascites. Also noted are an enlarged heart, gallstones, and an enlarged spleen. The report continues with a notation that all organs had a dark reddish-brown discoloration. There was marked iron deposition in the liver and heart consistent with advanced hemochromatosis.

Iron tests done the day Sam died showed Sam's percentage of saturation was 93 percent and his ferritin 99,465 ng/mL.

20

One of the First Documented U.S. Cases of Hemochromatosis

The Story of Jack Ritter

"Please, hold the plane for us!" Bonne Ritter shouted into the phone. "We have a medical emergency! I have to get my husband to Mayo Clinic; it's urgent!" she emphasized. "What is Mr. Ritter's problem?" asked the Philadelphia airport employee.

Nearly screaming, Bonne yelled back in response, "It's life or death! He has been given twenty-four hours to live. Please, I beg you, hold that plane!"

"I'm not trying to pry, Mrs. Ritter; we want to put a special attendant on duty if it would help."

Amid all the chaos, fear, and anxiety, here was a calm voice of a caring person offering a helping hand. Bonne explained the medical crisis the best she could under the circumstances. "I'll never forget her response," Bonne says, remembering that bitterly cold day in February 1968. "Drive carefully, we'll hold the plane."

These words quieted Bonne momentarily, allowing her to gather her thoughts. The Philadelphia Airport was fifty miles from the Ritters' home. Without the cooperation of the airport Jack surely would have died.

Twenty-year-old Jack Ritter was an accomplished Franklin & Marshall College basketball player. During a heated and competitive game against their rival team Dickinson College, Jack fell to the floor in what later would be determined a grand mal seizure. The team doctor, who had not seen the seizure but was familiar with such disorders, had carried Jack off the court. He suggested

Jack go home for a complete examination by the family doctor.

Jack was a welcome sight to his mother. She had been ill and appreciated his company. His seizure experience became somewhat overshadowed by his mother's prolonged illness. She was being treated for an enlarged heart; her skin was very dark—just like Jack's. Her eyelids were the same color as the dark circles beneath her eyes. When Jack was finally able to see the family doctor, he was diagnosed with a mild heart attack, caused by a condition possibly inherited from his mother.

The diagnosis didn't keep him out of World War II, however. Expecting a classification of Four-F everyone was surprised that the army accepted Jack. His new bride, Bonne, was certain Jack would never pass the physical exam. In boot camp formation Jack collapsed three different times, yet he went on to serve his country on both the European and Pacific Fronts without complaint.

Returning from war physically unscathed, Jack was greeted by his wife, Bonne. It was time to start building a new life. Within a year of his return, Jack and Bonne were expecting their first child, Tom.

One night, only three days before their third anniversary, Bonne was awakened by what she initially thought was an earthquake. The bed was shaking, and she heard noises she was too groggy to interpret. She rolled over toward Jack; his body was rigid. Bonne had witnessed seizures before, so she knew what was happening to her husband. Tom was only nine months old at the time. He slept in a crib in the same room as his parents and was awakened by these unfamiliar noises. Bonne remembers seeing Tom's tiny figure peering at her from the crib, and not knowing which one to comfort first. Her experiences as a schoolteacher had taught her to keep calm in a crisis. She gently held on to Jack so that he would not hurt himself, while she tried to diminish the look of fear in her child's eyes with soothing words of reassurance.

A new family doctor told the Ritters that Jack had probably just had a very bad nightmare. This was not uncommon among war veterans who often relived terrible war experiences in their dreams. It was 1947; the word *epilepsy* was never mentioned. Society thought it was disgraceful to be an epileptic. The Ritters referred to the experience using a word their family doctor had offered. Saying that Jack had convulsions seemed a bit less offensive than saying he had had an epileptic fit.

Later that year, Jack began to have joint pain and he continued to have seizures. The family doctor made several referrals to specialists, but the Ritters didn't know which doctor to see first— the psychiatrist, osteopath, or endocrinologist. The psychiatrist gained more out of an interview with Jack than the other way around. Jack's positive attitude and pleasant demeanor were not what this doctor expected to see. The osteopath offered that Bonne could use a good massage. She appeared tense while Jack seemed relaxed, accepting the events without complaint. It was the endocrinologist, however, who offered the greatest amount of torture. He suggested Jack needed his bile drained weekly.

Without a word of complaint, Jack submitted to the doctor's orders. His sweet nature and strong faith were obvious in the way he endured several difficult, some painful, procedures. Each week for months he lay with his head near the floor and his feet elevated on an exam table. A tube was run down Jack's throat to somewhere in his gut. He said nothing of the discomfort, though he gagged each time the tube filled with green-yellow liquid. Next came the spinal taps, too numerous to count, followed by an EKG and an EEG. Back then, there were no sophisticated MRIs or CT scans. Jack's EEG was performed with fine needles that are implanted into the skull. Each of the needles sank painfully into his skull. These electrodes imbedded in Jack's head would send messages to a device that resembled a lie detector.

As it turns out the EEG and EKG provided the first evidence of something tangible. Jack had an abnormality in the front-temporal lobe. He was prescribed Dilantin and phenobarbital. The physician concluded from the EKG that Jack had a prolapsed mitral value.

By now Jack was thirty. He had been seen by seven doctors and been in six different hospitals. It was only the beginning. For fifteen more years he continued to see the very best of physicians, including a specialist from London. The Ritters' lives revolved around medication schedules, paperwork from insurance companies, and trips to doctors.

Jack's attitude miraculously remained positive and he never complained even though he had cause to do so. He was beginning to feel weak and too fatigued to keep up his usual twelve to fourteen-hour workday. His skin was still dark; his seizures continued. He was hospitalized for blood poisoning. Joint pain, abdominal pain, and heart arrhythmia continued. Now his personality was changing. He was often confused or cross, immediately apologizing for his behavior afterward. Jack wanted to be a good husband and father; he would never intentionally hurt Bonne or Tom.

In 1965 Jack had five grand mal seizures in the same night, which led to a referral to a neurologist at Mayo Clinic. Three days in Mayo resulted in a diagnosis of epilepsy, possible due to an injury to the front left lobe of the brain. By now the Ritter family didn't fear the consequences of using the word *epilepsy*. Years of trying to keep this deep secret only added to the imagination of the neighborhood gossip-ring. Jack's medications were adjusted, changing the time of day taken; the daily dose was left the same.

This worked for nearly two years. The Ritter family and his many physicians assumed Jack's problems were all related to the epilepsy. They were wrong. That year, 1968, would prove just how wrong they all were.

Within a two-week period of time Jack lost forty-one pounds. He mentioned that his mouth was very dry. The family doctor said he thought Jack had become allergic to the Dilantin and instructed Bonne to discontinue the medication for a few days and see what happened. Bonne protested strongly, reminding the doctor that Jack had been on this drug for twenty years and stopping it abruptly might cause him to seize and never recover.

The doctor snapped back at her, "So, now, you're the physician!" Bonne took a deep breath, trying not to show her anger at such a demeaning remark. She quietly offered, "I have read about this medication and its precautions. I am simply concerned for my husband's well-being."

Numerous phone calls and an eventful trip to a dermatologist, who noted Jack's liver was enlarged, began the cascade of events that would finally lead to proper diagnosis.

At 11:00 A.M. Bonne heard her name over the classroom intercom. She had an emergency call in the office. Adrenaline shot through her body as she raced from her room into the office where her caller waited on hold. "Hello, this is Bonne Ritter," she choked out. The family doctor, the same one who had talked with her days earlier, was on the other end of the line. "Bonne, it's serious. Four different specialists have no idea what is wrong with Jack, but they agree on one thing, that you need to get him to Mayo Clinic today." Emphasis was placed on the word *today*. A roar in Bonne's head nearly drowned out the rest of the message that three of Jack's vital functions had shut down.

It took her exactly eleven minutes to convince the airport employee to hold the plane. She raced to get Jack and rushed to the airport, a fifty-mile ride, where the Ritters made the flight that would save Jack's life.

It was nearly 9:00 P.M. when the plane touched down in Rochester, Minnesota, home of the Mayo Clinic. To Bonne and Jack's surprise and delight there stood Dr. Frank Howard the neurologist, ready and waiting with his station wagon. His expression betrayed his attempt not to look shocked. It had been three years since he had last seen Jack. Once in the car, Dr. Howard instructed Bonne to turn on the dome light. Next he asked to see the palms of Jack's hands. Jack weakly turned toward the physician and offered his right hand with the palm upturned.

Bonne saw the doctor's shoulders rise as a result of a deep breath taken when Jack's palm obviously confirmed something he suspected. "I think they'll find hemochromatosis," said Dr. Howard. Neither of the Ritters had ever heard the word.

Jack was admitted to Methodist Hospital, where nine doctors soon surrounded his bed. They spoke in low tones consulting one another. Jack was semiconscious, drifting in and out of sleep. He was exhausted. One physician remarked that nearly all of Jack's body hair was gone. Another noted the dark skin, especially the lines in Jack's hands and closed eyelids. On the ninth day and sixteenth doctor, the Ritters were told Jack needed a liver biopsy. Dr. Frank Howard held Bonne's hand; his gentle clasp offered consolation in this moment when she was trying to understand what was happening. "You mean to tell me that after all he has been through, you need a biopsy to confirm what sixteen different doctors agree is hemochromatosis?"

"We could all be wrong, Mrs. Ritter," the doctor replied softly. Bonne was moved by the humbleness of the physician.

Undeniable proof was provided with the biopsy. Fortunately there was no cirrhosis, even though they said Jack's liver was so large it would fill a dishpan. It was a small miracle that there was no cirrhosis or cancer, considering the years of unchecked iron accumulation. Another shock as a result of the biopsy was that Jack had diabetes—a consequence of the hemochromatosis, the physician explained.

Bonne remembers being handed a sheet of paper with a single paragraph describing hemochromatosis. When she and Jack arrived home, the family physician had the same paragraph except that his included a line about prognosis. He informed Bonne that Jack probably had about nine months to live. Bonne called the doctor at Mayo who told her the prognosis depended upon how well Jack complied with therapy and followed his diet. At the time Jack was forty-six.

The next twenty-nine years would include meeting one of the finest physicians in the Reading, Pennsylvania, area, Dr. William Reifsnyder. With his help, Bonne saw her husband through excruciating arthritic pain, brittle diabetes, hip replacement surgery, numerous TIAs, and three heart attacks. In 1996 Jack was hospitalized with kidney failure.

Jack died September 19, 1996. He was seventy-three. Surviving twenty-nine years after his diagnosis, he remains one of the first documented cases of hemochromatosis in the United States. Always joyful and in good spirits, he was a model father, husband, and patient. He and Bonne had been married fifty-two years in August of that year. They celebrated in Jack's hospital room with a small cake and a coffee cup toast to their years together. She and Jack had talked about starting a support group for people with hemochromatosis. "Honey," he had said, "if we save one person from going through what we have gone through, it would be worth it."

Bonne carried on Jack's hope to help people. She has one of the best-attended HHC discussion groups in the United States. She and John Haille, who is mentioned in the treatment section of this book, participate along with Dr. William Reifsnyder, internist, and Dr. Marc Filstein, hematologist and head of the

Keystone Blood Bank. Besides the discussion group meetings, Bonne and her colleagues participate in health fairs speaking and distributing the Iron Disorders Institute's pamphlet "Diagnosing Hemochromatosis."

21

Two Brothers Spared Thanks to
One Sharp Physician

The Story of Cliff and Chris
After five physicians and ten years of trying to get a diagnosis, the suspense was unnerving. Dr. Craig Woodward glanced down at the lab results and looked up at his forty-year-old patient, Cliff, who was hopeful that this time he would hear something promising. Woodward had been recommended by one of Cliff's friends who was a nurse.

"You have a disease that is potentially fatal, if not caught in time," Dr. Woodward informed his patient. The words had not had time to sink in before Dr. Woodward continued, "And we caught it in time. You have hemochromatosis, an inherited disorder of iron metabolism."

Cliff asked for more information. "Your body absorbs more iron than people with normal iron metabolism. It's very treatable," Dr. Woodward explained. He had "caught it in time" because at the time, Smith/Kline Clinical Laboratories happened to include in its standard blood panel the tests that prompted the doctor to suspect and further test for hemochromatosis. Woodward was familiar with hemochromatosis and suspicious of Cliff's vague seemingly unrelated symptoms of joint pain, stomach problems, and elevated liver enzymes. When Dr. Woodward ordered an Executive Blood Panel, serum iron jumped out as abnormally high. Woodward knew the tests to do next, fasting transferrin iron saturation percentage and serum ferritin.

Cliff told Woodward that over the years, his unusual liver enzymes had been referred to as perhaps some type of low-grade/chronic hepatitis. "Based upon these findings, one doctor suggested I cut back on alcoholic beverages," Cliff continued. "I like a glass of wine with dinner now and then, but I certainly would not consider myself a drinker."

Cliff's joint pain was diagnosed as arthritis. He was given a prescription pain reliever. His bursitis was due to "too many bumps and bruises from an active lifestyle." Cliff loved water and snow skiing, cross-country motorcycling, surfing, tennis, touch football, and he had been in two automobile wrecks. Again, his pain reliever should help.

Cliff was told his stomach problems were most likely stress-related; his job as an Atlanta criminal prosecutor involved high-profile work, which was often nerve-racking. The doctor prescribed an antacid, which did not work. He was given Tagamet™.

Woodward listened attentively as Cliff continued the saga that led him to the present. "One doctor thought I had some illusive cancer. Another doctor noticed what appeared to be my year-round tan, except that I had no tan lines."

Dr. Woodward measured Cliff's iron saturation and ferritin. Both were elevated; though Cliff only recalls his ferritin was near 2,000. A cat scan of his liver helped confirm the HHC diagnosis. "No one considered my many ailments as symptoms of a single disease," Cliff adds. Dr. Woodward ordered therapeutic phlebotomy; Cliff went twice weekly at first, then once weekly. He reports that "the therapy has virtually eliminated my symptoms."

This physician's proper diagnosis of Cliff led to the diagnosis of Cliff's younger thirty-five-year-old brother Chris who, as it turns out, had a much more advanced case of hemochromatosis. Chris lived in the country where he drank iron-rich water and cooked in iron skillets. He too had complained of symptoms similar to his older brother Cliff, but never gave it thought there might be an inherited link. Chris's ferritin was 9,000 when first tested. He was seen and treated by another doctor other than Dr. Woodward, because he was eighty-five miles away.

At first Cliff's insurance would not pay for the phlebotomies, even though the cost was minimal. The Atlanta Red Cross in his area was not considered qualified to do therapeutic phlebotomy, but with the help of Dr. Woodward and cooperation of Red

Cross Director Dr. Grindon, this particular center now performs therapeutic phlebotomy at no charge.

Cliff concludes, "Thanks to the right factors being in place and coming to the attention of the right doctor, my family has been spared the tragedy of two brothers losing the battle to a potentially fatal disease. This is a battle that is needlessly being lost by others."

22
One Man's Advice

"DON'T WAIT LIKE I DID; IF YOUR DOCTOR
SUSPECTS THIS, GET ON IT, AND STAY WITH IT!"

—*Tug Nix*

Story of Tug Nix

Tug Nix spotted his medical chart; it was within reach. He grabbed the folder, returned to his seat, propped his right foot on his left knee, dropped the folder on his crossed leg, and flipped open the file. His rationale was that "I pay the doctor to make these files. I'm entitled to see what's in them." The receptionist for the Parkway Family Practice glanced at Tug and smiled. She noticed he had picked up his chart.

He scanned down through several unfamiliar words. Some words were too large to venture attempted pronunciation, but one popped out at him. It was ferritin.

"Woooowheeee." Was Tug's response to the numbers beside the word *ferritin*.

Dr. Hamilton came into the reception area in time to hear Tug's remark. He motioned for Tug to follow him to his office. "Your ferritin is 6,895; that's about 200 times more than normal. You have a saturation percentage of 96 percent. Tug, you really should have had that liver biopsy," Dr. Hamilton concluded.

"I suppose you're right, Doc. I should have kept that appointment last year when you sent me to the gastroenterologist," Tug confessed. "I'm ready now."

This had not been Tug's first visit to the Parkway Family Practice physician. One year earlier he had asked Dr. Hamilton if there was anything that could be done about his aching joints. Prior to finding Dr. Hamilton, Tug had suffered for more than fifteen years with painful joints. He had been to the Asheville Hand Center, since most of his pain was in the first two fingers of his hands. They had given him a prescription for pain medication, which Tug never filled. He took over-the-counter medications for pain, finally settling on Aleve. It worked to dull the pain, but nothing really made the searing ache go away entirely. Tug decided that the ache would become his constant, though annoying, companion.

An early morning phone call from Dr. Hamilton was a delightful surprise for Tug. "What in the world are you doing calling people at 6:30 in the morning?" he asked his doctor. "You need to come in right away; today if possible," was Dr. Hamilton's response. Tug complied.

Hamilton told him that his iron levels were elevated and he suspected a condition called hemochromatosis. He explained that hemochromatosis has as a consequence joint pain, diabetes, liver disease, and heart trouble. He went on to tell Tug that this was out of his field and that a liver biopsy was needed to confirm diagnosis. Tug winced; but he trusted Dr. Hamilton and goes on to describe him.

"Besides being a caring doctor, he is a gentleman, and an all-round good and kind man. If he says I need a liver biopsy, then I need one."

The first available appointment with the gastroenterologist was not for four months; Tug confirmed the time slot. He turned to his wife, Barbara, who was five months pregnant, and remarked, "My appointment is right at the time of your due date." An interesting observation, since their son John Tyler Nix decided to be born the same day as Tug's appointment with the gastroenterologist.

"I forgot everything!" Tug laughs. "Things were nuts; I didn't remember the appointment 'til weeks later. Then I just decided that high iron, so what? At least it isn't cancer. I actually thought it would just go away, like some disappearing act or something."

Tug's disregard for his iron levels allowed the metal to accumulate and add to his troubles. Excessive thirst and frequent trips to the bathroom at all hours of the day and night were also ignored. Tug was, however, scheduled to see a chiropractor, who checked his blood sugar levels. "My levels were sky-rocket high!" remembers Tug. The chiropractor advised Tug to get to Dr. Hamilton immediately. Hence the follow-up trip to Parkway Family Practice and the decision to keep the next appointment with the gastroenterologist.

Liver biopsy confirmed Dr. Hamilton's year-old suspicion. Therapeutic phlebotomy started immediately on an initial schedule of once a week. This wasn't aggressive enough; Tug's levels were not moving, and he asked for more frequent extraction. The gastroenterologist was hesitant to step up the frequency and told Tug so.

Tug Nix decided to get serious about this thing called hemochromatosis. He began to search for information. Among some of literature he found was Iron Disorders Institute's magazine and booklet describing therapy. "I read how the iron is pulled from ferritin to make new red blood cells. The IDI materials really inspired me to have another talk with my gastro-man," Tug comments.

After convincing the gastroenterologist that he could tolerate more frequent phlebotomy, his extraction schedule was increased to twice a week. Tug tells his experience with treatment. "My hemoglobin was checked before each blood draw. It was always 14.5 or 15.0. No other tests were done until I nearly collapsed in the doc's office one day. My hemoglobin was still normal but my ferritin was only 9. When I re-read the IDI materials I figured out I had been over-bled. Believe me, it was no picnic. I learned the true meaning of being tired. I was weak as a newborn kitten."

Between the physician and his straight-talking, take-charge patient named Tug Nix, they agreed, no phlebotomy for a couple of months. Two months later, Tug was feeling somewhat better. His hemoglobin was back up to 14.7. He continues his phlebotomy treatments monthly at Mission St. Joseph Hospital Outpatient Treatment Center in Asheville, NC, where he describes the service as "outstanding." Tug believes he feels better when his ferritin is in a range of 25–30 and will work for iron balance now that he is on the home stretch.

Tug says he has learned several things with this experience. When asked what he might say to help someone who might have hemochromatosis, he advises, "Don't wait like I did; if your doctor suspects this, get on it, and stay with it!"

When he is not rebuilding a diesel engine or telling someone they ought to donate blood, Tug takes to the western Carolina mountain roads on his "Henry"-Davidson, so named by his three-year-old son, John Taylor, who misheard the word *Harley*.

23

One More Reason To Stop Smoking

The Story of Two Swiss Children

On December 6, 1934, a forty-four-year-old mother of two was admitted to Hospital de La Chaux de Fords, Switzerland. She was experiencing shortness of breath and chest pain. Family history of illness was not unusual, but the attending physician found a nodule, which he determined to be cancerous; so, he removed it surgically. Shortly after the operation, the woman's condition worsened. She complained of pain in the left side of her chest; a lung tap produced over a liter of red liquid. Three weeks later, another tap produced a liter of yellow-reddish-brown fluid. Now feeble, barely able to breath, and with a faint heartbeat, the woman was admitted to the hospital. More lung taps were done, and tumor tissue was found in the fluid; she was diagnosed with metastasis of lung carcinoma—and died three weeks later.

Barely nine months after her death, her thirty-six-year-old brother was admitted to the same hospital for prolonged bronchitis. He was diagnosed with pleurisy. Four months later he returned to the hospital complaining of bronchial pain. An x-ray showed in the lower third of the right lung, directly above the diaphragm, a poorly defined shadow. He was treated, but developed a severe cough and eventually returned to the hospital. A pleuropuncture (tap) brought forth the same yellow-reddish-brown, cloudy liquid as that of his now deceased sister.

Fluid extracted from his lungs also contained tumor tissue; he was diagnosed with metastasis of a lung carcinoma—same as his sister. The patient was given radiotherapy, which seemed to have favorable effects.

Rarely had this doctor seen lung cancer in patients so young. The occurrence of lung cancer within relatively young individuals from the same family prompted the doctor to ask more detailed questions about the family's history. Conversations with the patient revealed that when he was a child, his mother worked at home polishing screws for a watch factory. She used a rotating steel disk onto which she continuously dusted a red polishing powder.

From their birth until the boy was twelve, and his sister

DID YOU KNOW ⁉️

The story of the Swiss brother and sister who died of lung cancer lay among papers in the office of Eugene Weinberg, Professor of Microbiology, Indiana University, for decades. The original 1936 document was published in German. Dr. Weinberg knew the basic contents of the story, because a colleague who spoke German translated the article for him. In 1998, David Garrison's German teacher Georgia Williams, Wade Hampton High School, Greenville, SC, translated the entire paper, and wrote the translation out in longhand, which was nine pages long. The handwritten words were so beautiful and precise, that this version remains the only known translation, just as she wrote it. The original paper and other scientific papers are used as reference material by Iron Disorders Institute.

twenty, both siblings were always in the room where the mother worked with this powder. Initially they were present as spectators, then as helpers. It followed that another sister had spent eight years away from the family. She was still in good health. The brother, however, now only thirty-six, died within a year following the death of his older sister. Curious, the physician contacted the watch factory and was told the powder was iron oxide. The doctor obtained a sample of the powder and had it analyzed to be certain. Indeed, the polishing dust contained the metal iron.

Both siblings had been exposed to prolonged inhalation of iron dust. That they died of lung cancer would be no surprise to someone who knows about hemochromatosis and iron overload. What may come as a surprise is that these children did not need to have hemochromatosis to have iron-loaded lungs.

In several research studies, mice and rats were exposed to ferric oxide-dust. In one report, lung tumors were observed to develop in one third of the iron-dusted mice as compared with one-tenth of animals who had inhaled iron-free dust. In another study, lung tumors occurred in 73 percent of rats exposed to respiratory ferric oxide, but no tumors in controls.

Tobacco plants accumulate a large quantity of iron in their leaves. A recent study reported as much as 60 million picograms of iron per cigarette. Mainstream tobacco smoke is estimated to contain as much as 0.1 percent of the metal contaminant; that is, 60,000 picograms of iron per cigarette smoked. Thus a one pack/day smoker could inhale over one million picograms of iron per day. In a number of reports, alveolar macrophages of smokers have been found to be brimming with iron—in most cases, in amounts sufficient to prevent the alveolar macrophages from killing cancer cells and pathogenic microbes. Additionally, both the gas and tar phases of cigarette smoke have been shown to dislodge iron from its ferritin receptacle and promote iron-dependent macrophage destruction. Accordingly, it is no wonder that moderate smokers have a ten-fold increased risk and heavy smokers a 15-25 fold increased risk of dying from lung cancer.

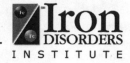

PART SIX

Taking Care of Yourself

"THERE ARE A NUMBER OF PREVENTIVE MEASURES A PERSON CAN USE TO SLOW DOWN IRON REACCUMULATION."

—John Beard, Professor of Nutrition,
Pennsylvania State University,
Iron Disorders Institute Scientific
Advisory Board Member

24

Individualizing Treatment

Treatment for iron loading conditions such as hemochromatosis is therapeutic phlebotomy, which is blood extraction. It is a relatively straightforward and simple procedure that can be done in a blood donation center, some physicians' offices, some university medical centers, and hospital therapeutic labs. The frequency of phlebotomy treatments and quantity of blood extracted may differ from patient to patient. Even the method of extraction can vary. Each case of hemochromatosis is different—unique in some way—and thus calls for individualized therapy.

Some factors that influence de-ironing include a person's age, weight, gender, general health, diet, and behavior such as tobacco and alcohol use, water consumption, medication, and compliance with therapy. Also, people with iron loading conditions such as hemochromatosis have different loading and unloading patterns.

Age: Young and elderly individuals confirmed to have iron overload warranting phlebotomy may not tolerate the standard blood extraction of 500cc twice a week. Further, it is unusual for someone younger than eighteen to need frequent or numerous therapeutic phlebotomies.

Weight: Individuals who weigh less than 110 pounds do not have the body mass to support standard extraction. For these individuals minimal therapeutic extraction or removal of 250–300 cc could be considered. This quantity also works well for the young or elderly. The treatment may need to be done more frequently depending upon iron levels.

Gender: Requirements for iron differ in males and females. A female body contains approximately 3.5 grams or 3,500 milligrams of iron; males contain about 4 grams or 4,000 milligrams of iron. This difference has more to do with average body mass than need, although a female's need for iron fluctuates more often than a male's. Pregnancy and menstruation affect iron needs, increasing demand and absorption of the metal significantly.

> "IN TWO LARGE SERIES OF SYMP-TOMATIC PATIENTS, THE YOUNGEST SUBJECTS WERE 18 AND 19 YEARS OLD. BASED ON THESE DATA, IT SEEMS WISE TO PROPOSE VENESECTION THERAPY FROM 18 YEARS OF AGE."
>
> —*EASL International Consensus Conference on HHC,* Journal of Hepatology *2000*

During the menstrual cycle a woman's natural iron regulatory system takes care to increase absorption of iron from her diet. Her normal absorption rate of one-half to 1 milligram is stepped up to 1.5–2 milligrams per day—the female body's natural response to blood loss. The average period lasts anywhere from two to five days. Blood loss during this time is estimated to be as little as 60–250 milliliters or about 2 tablespoons—a light period, to as much as 1 cup—a heavy period. A unit of blood, which is 450–500cc, extracted by phlebotomy is about one pint or two cups in volume and contains about 200–250 milligrams of iron.

Heavy menstrual flow might result in blood loss of one cup, about a 1/2 pint of blood per cycle, which contains about 100–125 mgs of iron. Females who still have regular menstruation can lose iron in this way, and be somewhat protected if they have an iron loading condition. When blood loss, and thus, iron loss, is greater than the body's ability to compensate, anemia develops.

> "RAPID MOBILIZATION OR REMOVAL OF IRON FROM YOUTHS OR ELDERLY MIGHT RESULT IN DAMAGE TO THE CONDUCTION SYSTEM OF THE HEART, AND CAUSE LIFE-THREATENING HEART ARRHYTHMIA, OR EVEN SUDDEN DEATH BY HEART ATTACK."
>
> —*IRON2000 USA Scientific Conference*

General health: When a patient is in relatively good health, treatment is a bit easier to establish, and maintenance can be

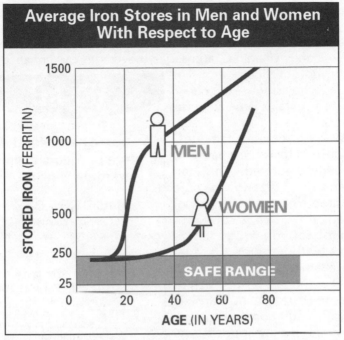

Average Iron Stores in Men and Women With Respect to Age

routine. If a patient's health is compromised, for example, by heart arrhythmia and the possibility of cardiac arrest, a physician might employ a combined approach. Less-frequent phlebotomy augmented by iron chelation therapy might offer a safer, albeit slower, method of de-ironing such a patient.

Iron chelation is the removal of metals, such as iron, pharmacologically by special chemicals that bind with the metal so that it can be excreted in urine. This type of chelation should not be confused with EDTA chelation, done by alternative clinicians. This type of chelation therapy does not remove iron, though it can remove other heavy metals from the blood stream. Health food store claims of oral products that remove heavy metals are misleading. Currently the only pharmacological iron chelating agents approved for use in humans are deferoxamine (also spelled desferioxamine), called DFO and sold as brand name Desferal, and an agent called deferiprone or L-1, sold as an oral iron chelator under the brand name Ferriprox.

Diet and Behavior: If a person smokes, drinks alcohol, and

consumes red meat frequently, these factors will hasten reloading and frequency of extractions may have to be increased. Red meat contains the kind of iron most highly available through diet. Alcohol, vitamin C, and sugary beverages can enhance the absorption of dietary iron. For those who smoke or chew, tobacco contains large amounts of iron.

Water: Adequate amounts are needed to assure a person is properly hydrated. This can mean the difference in time required to extract one unit of blood. Also, heavy consumption of soft drinks or sugary juices without drinking adequate amounts of water can affect some test results such as glucose (HbA_1c) and transferrin iron saturation percentage. These levels may appear to be higher than they actually are, causing a physician to order a phlebotomy that may not be needed.

MYTH

Some healthfood store products claim to remove iron...

INCORRECT

Over-the-counter oral remedies do not significantly remove iron from the body. Iron is removed through blood loss or special pharmaceuticals developed as chelators for this specific purpose.

Once a treatment frequency schedule has been established it is up to the patient to be compliant with therapy.

Compliance: A patient can be properly diagnosed and not comply with therapy. Frequently skipping phlebotomy treatments, or allowing too much time to lapse between getting de-ironed and the initial maintenance, can result in reaccumulation of iron. This might necessitate another round of therapeutic phlebotomies. Properly de-ironed patients who follow a donation schedule that controls iron levels should not have to repeat phlebotomies at a therapeutic rate.

There is no exact means of determining how much iron has accumulated in tissues. A physician can make fairly good estimates of phlebotomy frequency when taking into consideration all variables that are unique to a patient, such as the presence of liver disease or other inflammatory conditions. In confirmed iron overload, Ferritin is a good indicator of iron levels and can provide an approximation of the amount of iron to remove, but it is not necessary to retest ferritin often.

Using Ferritin to Estimate Phlebotomy Frequency
Ferritin does not need to be measured frequently. An initial serum ferritin can provide a physician with information that can help establish a rough estimate of the number of phlebotomies needed to reduce ferritin to a range where frequency of extraction might be changed. Each nanogram of ferritin represents 10 milligrams of mobilizable iron (the College of Pathology uses 7.5mg). A rough estimate of mobilizable iron and possible number of extractions can be made using a calculation of initial ferritin x 10. This calculation is not an exact science, and physicians or patients should not depend solely on the accuracy of such a calculation. Used as a starting point and with careful consideration given to hematocrit, a physician might be able to determine when ferritin levels have dropped low enough to reevaluate a patient's therapy regime.

Importance of Hemoglobin/Hematocrit
Hemoglobin/hematocrit will rebound or remain within normal range for patients who have iron overload. As blood is extracted, bone marrow is stimulated to make new red blood cells. Iron is required by these new red blood cells to make hemoglobin. So as blood is removed, new cells are made to replace those lost. Red blood cell production can keep up with making sufficient quantities to meet the body's needs, but it will not fully replace the huge quantity of red blood cells extracted. Eventually the body gets rid of excess iron while maintaining a healthy level of red blood cells and hemoglobin. When the patient's hematocrit reaches 34 percent on any one occasion, and there are no other complications such as internal blood loss or disease, the patient is likely de-ironed and can assume a maintenance program.

This is also a good time to retest serum ferritin, and transferrin iron saturation percentage. A rate of mobilization can be determined that will affect a person's maintenance program.

Take Care Not to Be Overbled

Sometimes a physician can forget to closely monitor a patient once initial phlebotomies are under way. For some patients phlebotomy schedules may be as often as twice a week for months. It is easy for a physician to lose track of this individual and, over time, the patient may continue to follow the same schedule of extraction when, in fact, they are overdue for reevaluation and a possible change in therapeutic frequency.

Forced-Sustained Anemia

It is still the practice of some physicians to bleed patients until hemoglobin remains at 10 g/dL or lower for a period of three weeks. This approach, forced-sustained anemia, may be an effective treatment and a tolerable approach for a thirty- or forty-year-old in relatively good overall health, but for many this practice is too extreme.

Methods that can lead to overbleeding and the development of prolonged iron deficiency anemia can result in trading one health problem for another. Of special concern are patients younger than twenty, females of any age, but especially those who are postmenopausal, and males older than fifty-five.

The practice of forced-sustained anemia is thought to be the only way to remove hemosiderin, an iron-containing compound. Excessive levels of hemosiderin can most definitely alter the function of vital organs and lead to disease. However, good studies provide that when ferritin reaches 10 ng/mL there is no detectable hemosiderin in the liver. Therefore bleeding repeatedly when ferritin levels have reached 10 ng/mL will offer no known benefit.

DID YOU KNOW

According to the College of American Pathologists

...red blood cell production is best challenged when hemoglobin values are 13.3g/dL or greater

Frequency of Extractions

Terms such as "aggressive phlebotomy," "routine extractions," "minimal or partial extraction" are used to define frequency of treatments. Generally, in any adults with very high levels of iron where serum ferritin is greater than 1,000 ng/mL with an accom-

Treatment Options

Treatment for iron overload in those who do not have concurrent anemia is therapeutic phlebotomy. Most patients are candidates for standard phlebotomy. **Patients should have a pretreatment spun hematocrit of > 34-36%.** Quantities removed by phlebotomy can vary from minimal extraction of 250cc up to large volume extraction of 600cc. Extraction continues until ferritin reaches 25ng/mL on one occasion so long as pretreatment HCT remains above 34%.

| | TYPE OF PHLEBOTOMY | | |
	STANDARD	MINIMAL VOLUME	LARGE VOLUME
Patient Profile	most patients	for juveniles, older or frail individuals and those with co-existent illness such as heart problems	unique cases such as adults with extremely high iron levels and other medical complications
Procedure	extracted from vein in the arm using 16 gauge needle (similar to routine blood donation)	extracted from vein in the arm using 20-22 gauge butterfly needle with vacuum bag	chest port surgically implanted near collar bone area
Duration of Procedure	15-20 minutes	15-20 minutes	15-20 minutes
Approx. Volume Blood Removed	450-500 cc of blood	250-300 cc of blood	600 cc of blood
Approx. Iron Removed	approx. 250 mg of iron	approx. 125 mg of iron	approx. 300 mg of iron
Frequency of Treatment	one or two times weekly	one or two times monthly	one or two times weekly
Important Notes	increasing the frequency to twice a week should be considered to facilitate more rapid iron depletion	frequency may be increased depending on patient tolerance patient may have small, inaccessible, scarred or rolling veins patient may be unable to tolerate standard volume of blood removal	serious procedure not to be considered a routine option

AVOID OVER-BLEEDING

panying transferrin iron saturation percentage greater than 55 percent, aggressive extraction is appropriate. Aggressive extraction is the removal of two units per week for an extended period of time.

Adults with moderately high ferritin but a levels that is below 1,000 ng/mL and an accompanying transferrin iron saturation percentage greater than 55 percent might also begin with aggressive phlebotomy for the initial period of therapy but slow to weekly extractions within a few months.

Adults with ferritin in a range of 450–650 ng/mL with an accompanying transferrin iron saturation percentage greater than 55 percent might begin with weekly extractions and move to moderate extraction or removal of a unit of blood every two weeks. If de-ironing is not successful they may have to switch back to weekly extractions.

And for some, monthly extraction might be a good starting point, especially for individuals who are diagnosed early and whose iron stores haven't yet reached a very high level.

> "OF 353 VENESECTED PATIENTS, DISAGREEMENTS OR PROBLEMS REPORTED INCLUDED 43 PERCENT HAD PROBLEMS WITH NEEDLE PUNCTURE, 63 PERCENT EXPERIENCED IMMEDIATE FATIGUE, AND 28 PERCENT FOUND THE TREATMENT TEDIOUS."
>
> —*EASL Consensus Conference on HHC,* Journal of Hepatology *2000*

The time frame for de-ironing is predicated on how rapidly a person unloads iron, and how quickly he or she reaccumulates the metal. Initially high iron levels for those who consume large amounts of red meat, drink more than moderate amounts of alcohol, and who smoke will not only be more difficult to de-iron, but these individuals will likely reload more quickly. It is possible that aggressive extraction may need to be reinstated if fewer extractions are not sufficient to keep pace with the patient's loading pattern.

Tolerance
Most people will tolerate phlebotomy without many side effects. Fatigue is the common problem reported.

During the final phases of de-ironing therapy, red blood cell production is not able to keep up sufficiently to sustain hemoglobin levels and anemia results. Some physicians use this state of anemia to signal that the patient is de-ironed. Some patients can tolerate a temporary state of anemia but many cannot. Older patients especially might have difficulty with this approach to de-ironing.

> "DE-IRONING IS COMPLETE WHEN FERRITIN REACHES 20 NG/ML ON ONE OCCASION THEN REMAINS IN A SAFE RANGE OF 25 NG/ML WITH AN ACCOMPANYING TRANSFERRIN SATURATION PERCENTAGE <30 PERCENT WHILE PRE-TREATMENT HEMATOCRIT REMAINS >34–36 PERCENT."
>
> —*Iron Disorders Institute*

Keep Good Records
Keeping good records during the entire treat-

ment process is strongly advised. People think they will remember details but they will not. A careful diary of events can be beneficial to any wellness program. Making notations about response to treatment can be significant in adjusting frequency and duration of therapy.

Maintenance
Once a patient is de-ironed, that individual may donate blood routinely as defined by the attending physician for optimum quality of health or may have periodic therapeutic phlebotomy by doctor's order.

Frequency of donation or therapeutic phlebotomy will depend upon the patient's personal health profile as observed by the patient and attending physician: age, weight, response to treatment, symptoms, rate of iron unloading, and general physical condition. This is a very good time to incorporate steps that can prevent reaccumulation of iron. Remember to donate blood in time; mark a calendar to remind yourself. Follow some of the simple guidelines outlined later in this section.

> "VENESECTION OF 400–500 ML WEEKLY IS CONDUCTED UNTIL FERRITIN IS <20-50uGL AND TRANSFERRIN SATURATION <30 PERCENT."
>
> —*EASL International Consensus Conference on HHC,* Journal of Hepatology *2000*

25

Therapeutic Phlebotomy Explained

A phlebotomy is a procedure used to remove blood from a person. It is the opposite of a transfusion, which is a way to give blood to a person. Phlebotomy is used to reduce iron levels in people who have excess iron in their bodies, such as people with hemochromatosis.

Excess iron in a person's body can cause damage to the liver, pancreas, pituitary, joints, and heart. As a result of this damage, one can develop cirrhosis of the liver, diabetes, impotence, infertility, depression, arthritis, and heart failure. Therefore, removing the excess iron as soon as possible is critical to prevention of chronic disease.

People can lose small amounts of iron by taking half an aspirin a day. But for those with serious iron buildup, phlebotomy is necessary because it is the most efficient means of removing iron. With each treatment about 250 milligrams (mgs) of iron are removed.

If tests indicate a person has iron overload, a doctor's prescription or an order is needed to obtain the phlebotomies. Usually an order is written for weekly or twice-weekly phlebotomies so long as spun hematocrit remains between 34 and 36 percent.

Hemoglobin carries oxygen to the body's tissues and carbon dioxide away from those same tissues. Hematocrit measures the volume or amount of hemoglobin contained in a person's blood. These two measures are most important during phlebotomy. If hemoglobin levels do not rebound after a phlebotomy, a person might not have an iron overload condition. Also, if hemoglobin is not measured prior to removal of blood a person could have a heart attack as a consequence of insufficient hemoglobin values.

Phlebotomies might be done at a blood donation center, as an outpatient in a hospital, or even in a doctor's office. A doctor may advise places that provide treatment. Consider convenience of location, cost to do the phlebotomy, and how responsive the center is to the situation.

Before the phlebotomy is done, hemoglobin and hematocrit will be checked. Usually centers have labs on-site; the results will be forwarded to the attending nurse. These preliminary numbers help assure that a patient does not become seriously anemic (not enough iron).

Patients may request a copy of lab work from the office manager in charge of records in the doctor's office. Obtaining lab results is highly recommended so that a journal may be compiled. Journals will become a valuable tool if a person has to move to another town or seek treatment from another doctor. Knowing about the disorder and understanding the diagnostic process helps to speed recovery and avoid future health setbacks. Patients may request a Personal Heath Profile (PHP) form through IDI's Patient Services. The PHP will help a patient keep track of important health data.

After the preliminary tests for hemoglobin and hematocrit are finished, a nurse prepares the patient for the phlebotomy. Blood pressure, temperature, and heart rate (pulse) are measured and recorded on a patient's medical chart for future reference. After being notified that hemoglobin/hematocrit levels are within a safe range, the nurse will prepare the patient's arm for blood extraction.

A latex band is tied around the upper part of the arm. This helps the vein to stand up. One may have to squeeze a soft rubber ball or make a fist several times to help the vein remain accessible. The nurse then swabs an iodine-based antiseptic on the vein and all around the area near the vein. This is to disinfect the area where the needle is to be inserted and to make certain bacteria do not get into the system during treatment.

A special needle is then inserted into the vein. One might feel a little pinch, but it lasts only a second. A piece of tape is placed over the needle to keep it stable; the patient just sits back and relaxes. Some like to bring a headset with earphones or a good book to read during treatment. While relaxing, the blood flows from the needle, into a tube, and then into the blood bag. The blood bag sits on a special scale that measures the weight of the blood.

When the bag is sufficiently filled, about one pint, the phlebotomy is complete. The speed with which the blood bag fills depends on the thickness/thinness of blood.

Drinking adequate amounts of water, at least six to eight glasses a day for two weeks before the phlebotomy will help.

Some may be finished in as few as ten minutes or as many as thirty; again, it depends on the vein, and thickness of blood. After the phlebotomy the nurse will remove the needle from the arm. A person may need to keep the area bandaged or apply mild pressure if bleeding continues.

> **MYTH**
>
> Removing one or two vials of blood from the arm is the same as a phlebotomy.
>
> **INCORRECT**
>
> *Standard therapeutic phlebotomy is the removal of approximately 450-500cc of blood or a full blood bag.*

Resting for about twenty minutes following therapy is a good idea. This is a precaution to ensure a person does not get weak, dizzy, or pass out. A snack is made available while a person rests; having something to eat following therapy is a good idea for those who have a tendency to get weak after an extraction.

Tips to Feel Better Between Treatments
Between phlebotomies, you might consider drinking at least six to eight glasses of water a day and taking daily vitamins. B complex vitamins, which include B_{12} and folic acid and extra vitamin E, can be especially beneficial. Water hydrates your cells, and these particular supplements provide important antioxidants and help to build red blood cells.

A doctor can advise the daily dose of these vitamins because the dosage will depend on one's general health, weight, and age. It is important not to overdo it with vitamins; there is no scientific proof that taking more than the recommended dose provides a greater benefit. Also, consuming large amounts of water prior to therapy is not wise; it may actually be harmful. Consuming water in large quantities too quickly can lead to water intoxication, a serious condition.

In years past, all HHC blood was discarded. As of August 1999 the Food and Drug Administration announced hemochromatotic blood safe for use with the exception of blood from those who visited the UK between 1980 and 1996 or who have lived in the UK (Great Britain) for more than six months. This is to protect the blood supply from possible contamination of Creutzfeldt-Jakob disease (mad cow disease). As of late 1999, guidelines for use of this blood have been written so that centers can apply for a variance to use HHC blood. Some centers, especially private blood donation centers have obtained their FDA variance and can now use hemochromatotic blood.

26

Treatment Options

Phlebotomy is the most efficient known therapy for most individuals with hemochromatosis/iron overload. The procedure is simple, relatively inexpensive, and most people tolerate the procedure well. In exceptional cases, depending upon the circumstances, options to standard phlebotomy might be considered by a physician.

Apheresis
The procedure is similar to blood donation, except that blood components such as platelets, white blood cells, red blood cells, and plasma are separated during the donation process. Also, this procedure takes a little longer than routine blood donation. Apheresis utilizes a computerized cell separator, which safely and automatically removes a specific component and returns the remaining components to the donor. A patient's hemoglobin is checked prior to apheresis just as it is in routine blood donation. Afterward, the donor reclines on a contour chair where a needle is inserted into a vein in the arm.

Red Blood Cell and Plasma (RBCP) apheresis donation is used as an option to routine phlebotomy. This allows donors to give full transfusion doses of red cells and plasma through the same process used to donate one component such as platelets. After the red cells and plasma are removed, the remaining fluids are returned to the donor. Donors lose a smaller amount of fluids through the RBCP process than through a regular whole blood donation. A saline solution is added to components returned to the donor.

According to Dr. James Smith, Oklahoma Blood Institute, "The advantage to apheresis over standard phlebotomy is that a standard unit of blood contains about 40 percent red blood cells. A unit removed by apheresis contains nearly 80 percent RBC." If one does the math, it becomes apparent that one apheresis treatment removes approximately double the iron, or an impressive 500 milligrams per treatment as compared with 250 milligrams. Though apheresis is more efficient than phlebotomy for iron removal, it is expensive and may not be affordable to many people.

Dr. Stephen Nightingale of the U.S. Department of Health and Human Services, and Dr. Mary Townsend, Medical Director, Coffee Memorial Blood Center, agree that apheresis can be considered by individuals with iron overload. Dr. Townsend points out that apheresis can be helpful for persons who live in rural areas and must travel long distances for treatment. These individuals can get the equivalent of two phlebotomies with one apheresis treatment.

For John Haille, "Apheresis can't be beat." After two years of repeated elevated levels of serum iron and eventually finding a physician who knew to test saturation percentage and ferritin, John was properly diagnosed with hemochromatosis. His saturation percentage was 91 percent and his ferritin level was over 1,000. Nearly two years earlier, a previous physician had seemed unimpressed by John's ferritin level of 690. A second test by the same physician didn't alarm him either; by this time John's ferritin was 1,092 and his TS was 58 percent. However, by this time the physician had heard of hemochromatosis and referred John to a hematologist, where he received his diagnosis and began phlebotomy treatments. Fifteen phlebotomies spread over nineteen months was not aggressive enough to reduce ferritin to a safe range. John began to look for alternatives. After reading about apheresis, he decided this was the therapy approach for him.

His physician wasn't certain John was correct but he took care to measure John's hematocrit prior to each treatment, which resulted in successful de-ironing. John's prescription read: "Two unit apheresis every two weeks until serum ferritin is lowered to 20 ng/mL or less as long as hematocrit remains greater than 35 percent and hgb remains within range of 14–18 g/dL." Additionally the physician ordered monthly serum iron, ferritin, and liver enzyme levels.

Three years later and upon being successfully de-ironed, John obtained genetic analysis and was found to be homozygous for C282Y. He concludes that his parents had to be carriers, as they never had symptoms of any disease. Afterward, John's brother Patrick was diagnosed with hemochromatosis by liver biopsy.

Apheresis is available in any blood center; however, it is not routinely offered as a treatment option for those with iron overload. Oklahoma Blood Institute and Reading Pennsylvania Hospital therapeutic laboratory are two centers known to be using apheresis specifically for the purposes of de-ironing. Anyone who is at least seventeen years of age, weighs at least 110 pounds, meets requirements for donation, and is willing to pay the difference in price for the procedure might consider apheresis as a treatment option.

Another approach using apheresis is offered at the Departments of Transfusion Medicine and Immunotherapy and Gastroenterology, Hospital de Clinicas, University of Buenos Aires School of Medicine, University Center for Diagnosis and Treatment of Hereditary Hemochromatosis, Buenos Aires, Argentina.

The purposes of this study were to evaluate the tolerance, efficacy, and safety of isovolemic erythrocytapheresis (EA) in nonanemic patients with hereditary hemochromatosis (HH), and to assess the usefulness of recombinant human erythropoietin (rHuEPO) associated with EA to reduce treatment duration.

In ten asymptomatic patients with serum ferritin >400 ng/mL, transferrin saturation greater than 50 percent, and elevated liver enzymes, erythrocytapheresis (EA) with recombinant human erythropoietin (rHuEPO) and folic acid was performed on ten patients with hemochromatosis who were not anemic. The results were that red cell indices (red blood cell count), serum ferritin, other iron metabolism parameters (serum iron, transferrin, and transferrin saturation), liver enzymes, and other laboratory data were considerably improved.

The group concluded that this method offers better results in less time than traditional phlebotomy and that EA with rHuEPO is an effective therapeutic alternative for patients with HH.

"This is very interesting, but expensive. You could probably remove an equivalent of ~ 3–4 pints of red blood cells at a time. I could see this being used for patients with cardiomyopathy, but it would also be associated with possible cardiac arrythmias, and would have to be done under very controlled conditions," says Dr. Barry Skikne of the Kansas University Department of Hematology and Bone Marrow Transplantation and IDI Scientific Advisory Board.

Chest Port
Patients with exceptionally high amounts of iron, usually confirmed by liver biopsy, might benefit from an implant or chest port. Chest port or central venous catheters are tubes threaded through the vein in the upper chest under the collarbone. Two types are commonly used: internal, which is surgically implanted under the skin, or external, where the entry site portion is visible outside the skin.

A phlebotomist who performs therapeutic phlebotomy is also qualified to remove blood through a port. Hemoglobin/hematocrit levels are measured prior to extraction just as with other types of blood extraction. Blood is extracted from the port through a tube leading into a vacuum bag or bottle. This type of bag/bottle is needed to suction the blood through the needle into a tube and into a blood bag. Vacuum bags or bottles hold the same amount of blood, one unit or 450–500 cc of blood, the same as a standard blood bag.

A saline solution is used to clean the port, followed by a heparin flush. Heparin is a blood thinner and used to prevent clotting, one of the problems of this device. Another problem with ports is that they can work their way out of the body and have to be replanted.

Ports are not considered routine method for therapeutic phlebotomy. These devices are generally used to give medication in cases where a patient requires large amounts of medicine that must be given often, such as in AIDS and cancer patients. However, this device can work well for some patients where iron levels are extremely high, especially when access to veins is impaired or difficult.

"I would run back to get another one!" exclaimed Jim Browne Sr. shortly after the removal of his chest port. After complications caused by phlebotomy, Jim, diagnosed with hemochromatosis, needed an alternative. His arms were bruised and painful; he was not going to be able to tolerate the twice-weekly blood extractions his high iron levels required. With a ferritin level over 1,800 ng/mL and transferrin iron saturation percentage above 60 percent, Jim's attending physician felt de-ironing had to be aggressive.

An ultrasound-guided liver biopsy confirmed Jim's hemochromatosis. Fortunately there was no cirrhosis, and cancer was ruled out, so the thought of repeated phlebotomy and anemia didn't sound too bad to him. After five extractions, however, Jim couldn't tolerate therapeutic phlebotomy; his doctor recommended a chest port.

Jim's overall experience with the port was very good. He found the port convenient and efficient, commenting that approximately 600 cc of blood were removed each time rather than the standard 450 cc. He had a unique problem in that his port worked its way out of his body and had to be removed. This was not painful as much as it was uncomfortable. Jim's physician removed the port, bandaged the area, and decided Jim was sufficiently de-ironed. So he did not insert a new port.

Itching and burning at the site were among Jim's complaints in addition to two other problems. One, a false drop in platelets, was traced to a heparin flush done before blood work rather than after. Blood for complete blood count (CBC) is drawn from the port; because it had been flushed with heparin prior to drawing blood needed to run the CBC, his platelet level readings were misleadingly low. Jim's second problem was that he had to deal with moderately severe anemia. His physician extracted blood until hemoglobin was 9.5 g/dL, which left Jim with uncomfortable symptoms: fatigue, sensitivity to cold, leg cramps, dizziness, heart arrhythmia, headache, and muscle weakness. He missed more work than usual, and he was not very good company to his family.

"I don't think I needed to be bled so aggressively toward the end," remarks Jim. "This was not so much because of the port," he adds, "but a belief my doctor held that anemia was a necessary part of the therapy. I'm not so sure I agree."

Chest ports require surgical implantation. This is a serious procedure and should be discussed at length with one's physician. Most people with iron overload are not candidates for this treatment option.

Minimal Extraction

Individuals who are frail, elderly, small (less than 110 pounds), or whose veins are scarred and not accessible might benefit from a smaller needle such as the butterfly needle. This type of needle is

Butterfly needle

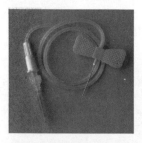

The smaller gauge needle makes insertion into the vein easier. Wings are pinched together to allow the phlebotomist a secure grip.

usually a 20–22 gauge as compared with a 16- to 18-gauge needle used for standard phlebotomy. Because the needle is smaller, removal of a standard unit of blood will take longer. Some individuals, such as those with heart conditions, especially arrhythmia, might not need a full unit removed, in which case minimal extraction or half-unit (250 cc) can be considered.

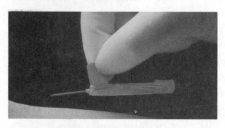

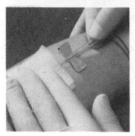

The needle is inserted into a vein in the arm and a connecting tube is attached to a blood bag.

Photographs courtesy of Becton Dickinson

Chelation Therapy

The type of chelation therapy used to de-iron patients who have iron overload should not be confused with EDTA (ethylenediame tetraacetic acid), a method used by some alternative medicine practitioners. EDTA is a broad-spectrum chelator, meaning that it binds with and removes a wide number of minerals. Therefore, it is not specific. In contrast, Desferal and deferiprone are highly specific for iron.

Iron chelation therapy is the removal of iron pharmacologically with an iron-chelating agent such as Desferal. Individuals who are transfusion-dependent or who have conditions where there is concurrent anemia with iron overload need chelation therapy to remove excess iron.

Desferal is not absorbed in the gut (intestinal tract); therefore, this drug must be administered intravenously or given by subcutaneous injection, using a portable battery-operated infusion pump.

Generally, the pump is worn at night, where slow infusion of the iron chelating agent is administered over a period of about eight hours for a duration of four to six nightly infusions per week. Patients might be given an additional 2 grams of Desferal intravenously for each unit of blood transfused. Desferal is injected separately from blood transfusions.

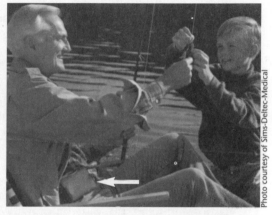

Photo courtesy of Sims-Deltec-Medical

Desferal is administered subcutaneously slowly at first, beginning with 1.0 gram, three to four times per week with monitoring of iron excretion in a cumulative 24-hour urine sample. If effective, the dose can then be adjusted upward, 1 gram at a time, up to four times per week, until the patient reaches a tolerable level. The dose should not exceed 50 milligrams/kg weight, or about 3 grams per day. Periodic examination of the patient is necessary until positive response to treatment is confirmed.

In the U.S., Desferal is currently the only drug approved for removal of iron by chelation. The drug is not very efficient, removing only about 6–10 mg of iron per treatment—compared with phlebotomy, which removes 250 mg per treatment. For this reason, Desferal is not appropriate for patients with hemochromatosis/iron overload. It is, however, currently the only treatment available to those who are transfusion-dependent. People with conditions such as thalassemia, some forms of leukemia, sideroblastic anemia, and myelodysplasia may need whole red blood cell transfusion to survive.

With every unit of blood, these patients are receiving approximately 250 milligrams of iron. With repeated transfusions, accumulation of iron occurs within one to one and a half years, and if a patient has complications such as leukemia, a complex treatment scenario is created.

Attending physicians will likely address the underlying cause of anemia first, before addressing iron overload. Desferal can then be administered to reduce iron levels after the primary condition causing anemia has been stabilized. For those with thalassemia major and who have been transfusion-dependent for a lifetime, chelation therapy should begin at the same time as transfusions.

Some physicians use a combination of Desferal and therapeutic phlebotomy, especially for patients with diabetic neuropathy and arthropathy. Dr. Paul Cutler of Buffalo, NY, reports this combination therapy results in a 50 percent increased improvement over standard phlebotomy alone. Individuals with cardiac involvement might benefit from the combination of Desferal and phlebotomy.

However, anyone with severe kidney damage is not a candidate for this type of treatment, as Desferal is not only excreted via bile and feces, but also via urine. Women who are pregnant, nursing, and children younger than three are not candidates for Desferal. It is not known how much of the drug gets into breast milk; thus, a mother who is receiving Desferal treatment might consider low-iron soy formula substitutes.

Immediate symptoms of adverse reaction to Desferal chelation therapy might include: visual disturbances, blurred vision, rash or hives, itching, vomiting, diarrhea, stomach or leg cramps, fever, rapid heart beat, hypotension (low blood pressure), dizziness, anaphylactic shock, and pain or swelling at site of intravenous entry. Long-term problems might include kidney or liver damage, loss of hearing, or cataracts.

Patients should report such symptoms immediately to their physician, who can adjust dosage. Further, physicians might examine a patient's visual status with slit-lamp fundoscopy (means of examining the eye) and his hearing status with audiometry or a hearing test. Liver enzymes (ALT, AST, GGT and

ALP), a kidney function test such as BUN, serum ferritin, and transferrin iron saturation percentage might also be measured by the attending physician.

Oral Chelators
A pill that can remove iron is high on the list of requests made by patients with iron overload. Initially produced to treat patients with thalassemia major, deferiprone (L1) is unique in that it is effective when taken orally. It is, however, a highly controversial drug. Dr. Nancy Olivieri at Toronto's Hospital for Sick Children studied deferiprone to determine its efficacy and efficiency. She concluded that the drug was more efficient than deferrioxamine (Desferal) in the first few days of application, but when used for periods longer than two weeks, the outcome for the patient was poor. Dr. Olivieri halted clinical trials of deferriprone L1. Halting a study is uncommon, except perhaps when there is a concern regarding safety of participants. Apotex, manufacturer of deferiprone, sought another source in Europe for trials needed to study the drug for use in humans.

In August of 1999, Apotex Inc.'s Ferriprox (deferiprone) was approved in Europe by the European Agency for the Evaluation of Medicinal Products for treatment of iron overload in patients with thalassemia when deferoxamine therapy is contraindicated or in those who develop serious toxicity with deferoxamine therapy.

Ferriprox is not appropriate for use by those who can tolerate phlebotomy.

Companies working to perfect oral chelators include:
- SunPharm Corporation (Geltex), Ponte Vedra Beach, Florida. Product name: HBED.
- Biomedical Frontiers, Minneapolis, Minnesota. Product name: HES-DFO.
- Norvartis Pharmaceuticals, Basel, Switzerland. Product name: ICL670A.

Future Technology
While laboratories around the world work to perfect additional oral chelators, a California-based company may have a novel approach to standard Desferal chelation therapy. Aethlon Medical, Inc., has obtained a U.S. patent on equipment that is designed to

remove metals such as iron from the body.

The equipment is called a Hemopurifyer and uses a hollow fiber device with immobilized desferioxamine (DFO). This device is a cartridge that can fit into any conventional dialysis machine.

Supported with funding from the National Institutes of Health, inventor Dr. Clara Ambrus, Buffalo General Hospital, and her colleagues, began studies to determine the efficacy (does it do what it is supposed to do?) and efficiency (does it do it well?) of the cartridge to remove the metal aluminum from patients with end-stage renal disease. Dr. Ambrus obtained FDA approval to test for the removal of aluminum along with additional FDA approval to test her novel design's ability to remove iron, lead, and platinum, which can be a byproduct of certain types of chemotherapy drugs.

Usually DFO is administered directly into the bloodstream intravenously, where it binds with iron and the iron is excreted in urine. Using the device, blood is treated with a circulation system similar to ones used in hemodialysis (kidney dialysis). Blood is extracted from the patient and mixed with DFO extra-corporeally (outside the body); DFO binds with iron contained in red blood cells and free iron in serum. Blood components are separated in a similar way used in dialysis or apheresis, returning platelets, serum, and red blood cells, along with a saline solution, back to the patient.

Because the chelation process takes place outside the body, none of the chemical gets into the patient's system, thereby eliminating side effects caused by DFO given intravenously (IV). The cartridge removes about 10 milligrams of iron per hour as compared with the IV DFO method where 3–4 milligrams per hour are removed. There are drawbacks; the cartridge must be used with standard dialysis equipment, which is not portable. However, the cartridge is designed to fit any dialysis machine including portable models when these become available.

Scientific data about the novel procedure and equipment have been examined by Iron Disorders Institute Scientific Advisory Board Members. Response has been mixed but promising. Most agreed that if Aethlon has indeed perfected a safe, effective, novel approach to chelation therapy, patients with concurrent anemia and iron overload will have a fairly significant alternative to standard DFO chelation. Benefiting from this new therapy can include individuals with transfusion-dependent iron overload, and specifically those with thalassemia major, sideroblastic anemia, aplastic anemia, and perhaps some forms of leukemia and MDS.

In Conclusion
Some individuals with iron overload will seek an approach to therapy that is less tedious than routine phlebotomy. In doing so they might be misled by some heavily marketed products claiming to remove iron. To date, for those who can tolerate routine phlebotomy, there is no other known method that is both more efficient and cost effective for the safe removal of iron from the body than this procedure. Individuals with iron overload who are considering therapy options are encouraged to:
- seek information about therapy from reliable sources such as respected scientific journals; read as much about a new therapy as possible
- make no hasty decisions about the therapeutic course of action, and
- discuss therapy options in detail with a qualified physician.

27

Why Is the Blood Thrown Away?

In April of 1999 when the Advisory Committee on Blood Safety and Availability unanimously concluded that blood obtained from those with hemochromatosis posed no greater risk than blood obtained from routine donors, patients with HHC across the USA rejoiced. Many patients with HHC were already donating regularly, but they had to watch helplessly as their blood was discarded as unfit for use. When the committee made its recommendation, we thought a long and wasteful practice had been stopped. Those of us present when the recommendation was made applauded the FDA for its decisiveness. Secretary of Health Donna Shalala's prompt response to the committee's recommendation that HHC blood was safe for use contributed to the groundswell of excitement.

One year later, however, HHC blood is still not accepted by many blood centers. Further, some blood centers seemed unimpressed by the matter. What happened to momentum? Providing us with answers is Dr. Mary Townsend, Medical Director, Coffee Memorial Blood Center and America's Blood Centers Chair of the Scientific, Medical, and Technical Committee on blood availability.

At the IRON2000 USA Scientific Conference in Arlington, VA, Dr. Townsend's presentation helped us to better understand the barriers still remaining that impede use of HHC blood. "Everyone wants to cooperate," she began, "but there are complications. Many private blood centers want the blood but they can't just begin taking it without going through major operational changes."

First, a center must apply for an FDA variance-21 CFR 640.3 (d) and 21 CFR 640.3 (f), to be precise.

The variance does not come without conditions. Though at present the FDA considers HHC blood safe for use, the FDA must be accountable to members of the public who receive this blood. Therefore it is only prudent for the FDA to ask for additional data as a condition of any center permitted an FDA variance. It is important to keep in mind that blood banking systems were designed to manage a public commodity that above all must be safe for use. The FDA's recommendation could have included HHC blood be labeled—a deterrent for use by anyone who knows little about iron. Extra data gathering seemed a small price to pay to gain access to such a rich resource of blood; centers are willing to comply, but it takes manpower and time to do the extra record keeping.

"That's not the only problem," Dr. Townsend adds. "Let's say a center applies for and receives a variance. That is the easy part; now they are tasked with rewriting standard operating procedures for donor qualification. Medical history, reasons for deferral, and testing procedures need to be changed. Therapeutic phlebotomy algorithms (process and order of procedures) have to be written and included; blood center employees have to be trained," she continues. "Further, some HHC donors need to donate as often as twice a week. Computer systems are not set up to track this level of frequency."

> ## FDA VARIANCE
> ### 21 CFR 640.3(d) and 21 CFR 640.3(f)
>
> Blood donors with HHC are subject to the same suitability requirements as are allogeneic donors, except for the time interval since the previous donation. Donations more frequent than every 8 weeks will be prescribed by a referring physician, or, for self-referred donors, by a blood center physician after examination and certification of health on the day of donation.
>
> Blood and blood components from donors with HHC, who meet all suitability requirements, may be labeled as suitable for transfusion and distributed as allogeneic units, without special disease state labeling. Blood collected from HHC donors who fail to meet any of the current suitability requirements will be discarded.

"It's not just a matter of hiring someone to rewrite the software," comments Gregory Hart, Director Georgia—The Blood Conection, Greenville, S.C. "Computer software programs that blood centers use must be approved by the FDA."

Of 75 centers sent a questionnaire about the issue of applying for the FDA variance 45 responded. Sixteen private centers have applied, 2 are not sure, and 27 do not intend to apply. Reasons given were varied. Some centers felt they were too small and did not have the funds to restructure themselves or to hire additional manpower to handle the added work. Some local hospitals continue to refuse to use HHC blood, so why go through the expense and time to restructure when the local demand for this blood is nonexistent? Also, some centers don't draw therapeutics, and some just want to wait for more information based on experience. Their well-entrenched concern for safety in the blood supply seems the key drawback to application for a variance and use of HHC blood. A person with HHC is perceived as having a potentially life-threatening disorder that requires blood extraction.

"Education is key," says Dr. Townsend. "Without significant education, it will never be understood that HHC is not a blood disease but a disorder of metabolism.

"People need to understand, there is no more iron in a unit of blood drawn from someone with HHC than there is in a unit of blood drawn from a non-HHC donor. Iron in individuals with HHC remains in their tissues and can only be removed 250 milligrams at a time per unit of blood—the same as anyone else who is donating."

Reasons Given Not To Apply For Variance (OR TO WAIT)
■ Don't draw therapeutics; or very few donors locally
■ No interested donors locally
■ HHC donors are already drawn after unloading (3)
■ HHC already drawn free (3)
■ Additional manpower needed to track
■ Confidentiality issues
■ Concerns over release of inappropriate units
■ Informed Consent concerns
■ Expensive to implement
■ Loss of income
■ Concern over infectious disease markers; what if it turns out there is a higher rate of reactivity and units are already transfused
■ Local hospitals will not accept
■ Low priority with all the other issues we are tackling now
■ Waiting for other centers

It is clear that individuals with HHC have a valid complaint when they see their blood discarded. It is also clear that the Department of Health and Human Services and many blood centers see this as a waste of a precious resource and wish to see the blood used. With adequate time, education, and appreciation on the part of both sides, the blood issue will likely correct itself. Meanwhile, there are ways you can help.

28

Keeping Iron in Balance with Diet and Preventive Measures

"AMONG 2,851 PARTICIPANTS, FOLLOWING DIAGNOSIS OF HHC,
65 PERCENT WERE TOLD TO AVOID IRON SUPPLEMENTS,
38 PERCENT WERE TOLD TO EAT LESS IRON-RICH FOODS,
27 PERCENT WERE GIVEN NO DIET ADVICE."

—*1996 CDC HHC Patient Survey*

What diet do I follow? is one of the most frequently asked questions by people when diagnosed with hemochromatosis.

"People want to know about diet," says Kay Owen, Manager of Patient Services, Iron Disorders Institute. "Individuals with hemochromatosis (iron overload) are concerned they will have to give up their favorite foods and are surprised to learn this is not always necessary."

A balanced diet of good lean meats, fruits, vegetables, and grains that are not heavily fortified with iron, along with a few practical measures, can help a person keep iron levels under control. The Nutritional Labeling and Education Act of 1990 (NLEA) provides for the nutritional content to appear on all food products in the United States. These panels are quite accessible, and helpful when initially setting up a diet plan for a person with an iron loading disorder such as hemochromatosis. What must be kept in mind is the difference in the type of iron contained in food.

Additive Iron

Additive iron found in prescription iron pills, most supplements, and fortified foods is inorganic, which means it is not derived from a living source such as vegetables or animals. Inorganic iron is in mineral form and is used to fortify foods. When in mineral form iron is ferric. It has to be changed to ferrous form to be absorbed by the body. Our body does this naturally with stomach acid, otherwise called hydrochloric acid or HCL, and later on in the small intestine with specific enzymes called reductases.

Previously, when iron was added to cereals and breads, it was in the form of iron filings. Food manufacturers have discontinued this practice, selecting ferrous sulfate or reduced iron to fortify these foods.

Other additive iron compounds one might see listed among nutrition information contained on food products include ferrous fumarate, ferrous gluconate, and iron-polysaccharide.

Two iron compounds, ferrochel and Fe-EDTA, are making their way into the marketplace as candidates for fortification by major food manufacturers. Individuals with conditions such as hemochromatosis that result in iron overload will need to avoid such fortified food products. These two additives have been found to exceed absorption capabilities of the commonly used ferrous sulfate.

Ferrochel is an iron bis-glycine chelate. Glycine is a nonessential amino acid used as a chelate. This chelate has a 2:1 ratio to the mineral, hence, "bis" meaning two glycines to one iron atom. Albion Laboratories, Salt Lake City, Utah, owns the patent rights to produce these type of chelates, which are much more effective at delivering a high bioavailable form of iron.

Fe-EDTA is a compound of iron salts and EDTA (ethylenediaminetetra-acetic acid), which is a broad-spectrum chelate, meaning it binds with many minerals. It, too, has performed well in the same absorption studies. Both EDTA and bis-glycine chelated iron were absorbed at the rate of two to three times that of ferrous sulfate. When combined with phytase, the enzyme that breaks down phytates in fiber, Ferrochel and EDTA increase the bioavailability of iron even more.

What is alarming about these super additives is that they are highly effective at overriding the normal iron regulatory mechanism. Persons with an undetected iron loading condition who consume products fortified with these super additives can accelerate iron accumulation and hasten organ damage.

Iron Absorption in Humans from Four Different Breakfasts When Fortified			
Basal	Basal + 3mgs Ferrous Sulfate	Basal + 3mgs Ferrochel	Basal + 3mgs Fe-EDTA
3.0%	5.3%	10.8%	14.9%

Iron Absorption in Humans from Four Different Breakfasts When Fortified *Plus Phytase*			
Basal	Basal + Ferrochel	Basal + Ferrous Sulfate + Phytase	Basal + Ferrochel + Phytase
5.1%	7.9%	10.1%	13.2%

Genetically modified foods are of equal concern for the same reasons. Japanese and Swiss scientists have successfully modified rice genetically so that it has increased iron.

Dietary Iron: Heme and Non-heme Iron
Dietary iron is organic, that is, derived from plants and animals. Plant-based iron is the greatest source of non-heme iron; plants actually contain heme iron, too, but in insignificant amounts. When we eat fruits, nuts, vegetables, and grains we are consuming non-heme iron.

The best source of heme iron is animal-based, although meat also contains non-heme iron. Heme iron is in a form that is easily absorbed by the body. Non-heme iron must first be reduced before it can be absorbed. Plant-based or non-heme iron is not the best source of dietary iron; however, when fortified, this type of iron can have a significant impact on the amount of iron that gets into the system.

When a person eats meat, especially red meat, they are consuming the flesh of the animal, which contains both hemoglobin in blood, and myoglobin in muscles. Hemoglobin and myoglobin contain iron in a porphyrin form, which is readily absorbed by the body.

Besides Australians and Argentineans, Americans are among the highest per-capita beef consumers in the world. There are no correlating heart attack figures for these three countries. However, according to the American Heart Association, National Centers for Chronic Disease Control and Prevention, and the World Health Organization, heart failure in these three countries was the second or third leading cause of death.

This is not meant to suggest that meat should be eliminated from one's diet, but to illustrate that by diversifying one's meat choices and eating red meat less often, there could be a significant preventive disease benefit as a result.

Bioavailability

Bioavailability is the degree to which a nutrient is available to the body for its intended use. Spinach, touted to be high in iron by the well-known cartoon character Popeye the sailor, has only about one milligram of iron per serving. Spinach contains oxalates, which impede iron from being absorbed, making the bioavailability of iron contained in spinach almost nonexistent. According to nutrient bioavailability expert Dr. Raymond Glahn, USDA, Agricultural Research Center, U.S. Plant, Soil, and Nutrition Laboratory, Cornell University, "What little iron one gets from eating spinach comes mostly from soil that clings to the leaves."

For humans, the best source of highly bioavailable iron is in meat, especially red meat. Fruits, vegetables, nuts, and grains contain a type of iron not readily absorbed, and iron supplements for those who do not need them are just aggravating a person's gastrointestinal system.

Over the years, bioavailability of nutrients such as iron has been somewhat of a mystery. Thanks to the Nutritional Labeling and Education Act of 1990 (NLEA), consumers can read from these labels the amount of iron in an ounce of meat, a gram of cereal, an egg, or a cup of spinach. But how readily we humans absorb iron contained in certain foods still depends on how available these foods are to the body.

In past years, the only way to determine iron absorption was through expensive animal and human feeding trials. This type of testing is called in vivo or in life. In vivo testing requires nutrients such as iron to be radiolabeled so they can be measured as they pass through the digestive tract and are absorbed.

Radiolabeling of the iron usually requires that a small, non-hazardous amount of radioactive iron be added to the food. The radiolabeled test nutrient contained in urine or fecal matter provides an indication of how much absorption took place. Measuring the amount of radiolabeled iron retained in the body indicates how much iron absorption took place. Although simple in concept, in vivo testing is time-consuming and expensive, plus one must make the assumption that the radiolabeled iron is absorbed to the same extent as the non-radiolabeled iron present in the food.

An "artificial gut" was invented by a team of U.S. Agricultural Research Service scientists at the U.S. Plant, Soil, and Nutrition Laboratory in Ithaca, NY. Dr. Raymond Glahn, a leading scientist on the Agricultural Research Team, notes that "this in vitro (artificial environment) model is unique because it couples simulated food digestion with a human intestinal cell line called Caco-2." Dr. Glahn points out that "the cost of using the assay (test) system will be only 20 percent or even less as compared with the cost of animal or human trials."

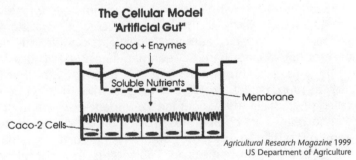

The Cellular Model
"Artificial Gut"

Food + Enzymes

Soluble Nutrients

Membrane

Caco-2 Cells

Agricultural Research Magazine 1999
US Department of Agriculture

The system is described in the diagram and thus far has been used to investigate iron availability from rice cereal, infant formulas, and iron supplements. Dr. Glahn states that the model "was validated by reproducing effects similar to those consistently observed in human studies." He believes that eventually the model will be used to measure bioavailability of other micronutrients such as vitamin A, zinc, selenium, and iodine.

"One of the results obtained thus far indicates that the high level of citric acid in bovine milk decreases iron availability in infant formula made with cow's milk," reports Glahn. Additionally, Dr. Glahn observed that apple juice contains one or more substances that offset the ability of vitamin C to enhance iron availability in infant rice cereal. Glahn believes that eventual isolation of these substances might lead to development of new classes of oral compounds that could prevent alimentary iron loading. Such compounds could be extremely valuable in slowing the rate of disease and death in millions of persons who are prone to absorbing excessive amounts of iron such as individuals with hemochromatosis. Further, this information can be extremely helpful for those who are iron deficient and who can correct deficiencies with iron-rich diets.

Effects of Foods and Food Products on the Absorption of Iron
There is no known agent that will impede the absorption of heme iron. However, besides oxalates, there are a number of food items that will impede absorption of non-heme iron by as much as 50 to 60 percent and in some cases up to 90 percent.

Foods and Food Products That Impede Absorption
Phytates found in whole grains, tannins in teas and coffees, phosphates in dairy foods, antacids, calcium supplements, antibiotics, citric acid, and apple juice can significantly reduce the amount of plant-based or non-heme iron one absorbs.

Phytates are compounds found in plants. High-fiber foods such as bran, cereal, beans, and peas are high in phytates. Also called phytic acid, these compounds impede absorption of iron.

Phosphates are compounds used to whiten products ranging from toothpaste to milk. They also have the ability to inhibit the absorption of non-heme iron. Food items that contain phosphates include bacon and ham, baking powder, cereals, milk products, cheeses, frozen fish, frozen potatoes, hot cocoa mix, puddings, marshmallows, sugar, and yeast.

Antacids and calcium supplements change the pH of the stomach, reducing the effectiveness of HCL.

Antibiotics: Desferal, a chelator given intravenously to individuals with concurrent iron overload and anemia, was initially developed as an antibiotic. It was learned in clinical trials that Desferal was ineffective as an antiobiotic but capable of binding with iron. Many antiobiotics seem to have this characteristic.

Apple juice: In a study to determine iron availability in infant cereal, Dr. Raymond Glahn of the USDA Agricultural Research Service notes, "Our findings suggest apple juice contains one or more substances that offset the vitamins' beneficial effects on iron uptake."

Oxalates: Contained in foods such as spinach, oxalates impede the absorption of iron.

Tannins, also called polyphenols, are compounds found in teas, such as orange pekoe and black teas, coffee, and red wines. Tannins have demonstrated the ability to inhibit absorption of non-heme iron. In studies conducted to test how well tannins in certain coffees performed, regular perked or dripped American coffees did not significantly inhibit iron absorption as much as espresso, instant coffees, and

BREAKFAST	
PHYTATE-RICH FOODS	Phytic acid content percentage of dry weight
Excellent	
Wheat bran cereals like All-Bran	3.0-5.0%
Oatmeal	2.4%
Raisin bran	1.8%
Good	
Shredded wheat	1.5%
Rye bread 0.8-1.5%	
Whole wheat bread	0.6-1.0%
Special K	0.7%
Product 19	0.5%
Poor	
Rice Krispies	0.24%
Pumpernickel bread	0.16%
White bread or French bread	0.03-0.13%
Cornflakes	0.05%
Raisin bread	0.09%

LUNCH, DINNER, and SNACKS	
PHYTATE-RICH FOODS	Phytic acid content percentage of dry weight
Excellent	
Lima beans	0.9-2.5%
Wild rice	2.2%
Red kidney beans	1.2-2.1%
Pinto beans	0.6-2.0%
Navy beans	1.8%
Good	
Rye bread	0.8-1.5%
Corn bread	1.4%
Soybeans	1.4%
Peas	0.9-1.2%
Whole wheat bread	0.6-1.0%
Barley	1.0%
Brown rice	0.9%
Corn	0.9%
SNACKS OR CONDIMENTS (SEEDS AND NUTS)	
Excellent choices	
Sesame seeds	5.3%
Pumpkin seeds	4.3%
Sunflower seeds	1.9%
Peanuts	1.9%

teas. The latter were the most effective, impeding up to as much as 90 percent absorption of non-heme iron when consumed with a meal. None of these beverages were effective when taken one hour prior to a meal; however, when taken one hour after a meal, their ability to impede iron absorption was as great as when consumed at the same time as the meal.

Iron Absorption in Humans from Four Different Breakfasts Containing Coffee/Tea			
Basal	Basal + American Coffee	Basal + Espresso	Basal + Tea
7.5%	6.7%	3.9%	3.9%

Foods and Food Products That Enhance Iron Absorption
Alcohol: Alcohol enhances absorption of iron and contributes to liver disease. Limiting alcohol consumption to social events and special occasions such as dining out or celebrations may help a person reduce the amount consumed. Studies show that heavy drinkers have high iron levels. Approximately 20 to 30 percent of those who are heavy consumers of alcohol acquire up to twice the amount of dietary iron as do moderate or light drinkers. Alcohol will hasten liver disease such as cirrhosis. Patients who have developed cirrhosis increase their chance of developing liver cancer by two hundredfold. Alcohol in the presence of high iron can also cause brain damage. Brains of alcohol-induced lab rats were found to have an alarming amount of "free iron" in the cells of their brains. A standard drink is defined as 13.5 grams of alcohol, 12 oz. beer, 5 oz. wine, 1.5 oz. distilled spirits. Moderate consumption is defined as two drinks per day for an adult male or one drink per day for females or those older than sixty-five regardless of gender. Options to consider might be nonalcoholic or low alcohol content beer and wine.

Vitamin C: Vitamin C binds with iron in a way that makes it highly bioavailable. Beverages fortified with vitamin C or naturally high in vitamin C such as some juices and vitamin C supplements are best consumed between meals with a snack. Limit vitamin C daily supplements to 200 milligrams or less. This nutrient is absolutely required for proper synthesis of collagen; however, vitamin C enhances absorption of iron, and its presence can contribute to iron's free radical activities. Avoid vitamin C–rich juices or C supplements seventy-two hours prior to testing iron levels, which can be altered by this nutrient. Substitute apple juice for orange or other C-rich juices taken at breakfast. Apple juice is thought to impede absorption of iron. Take supplements with low-iron meals or two hours before or after consuming meats.

Warnings, Dangerous Combinations, and Good Common Sense
Individuals with high iron levels increase their risk of infectious disease, such as viral hepatitis and bacterial infections. The following measures can protect a person who has an iron loading condition against unnecessary disease and prevent further organ damage by managing iron levels.

Tobacco: Tobacco products contain high amounts of iron. Not only does tobacco use rob your body of oxygen, but it also has an increased advantage of harming your health over other foods that contain iron. When foods or food products containing iron are eaten, the amount of iron absorbed from these foods is regulated in the intestine. When iron is inhaled, it bypasses this regulatory step; thus, iron contained in the tobacco smoke goes directly into the lungs. Also, any opportunity to impede absorption of iron, such as with phytates or tea, is lost. Inhaled iron collects in lung cells called alveolar macrophages. These are the cells that help fight against infections and cancers in the lungs. When heavily burdened with iron, these cells cannot protect a person against opportunistic disease such as Legionnaires' pneumonia. Also, cancer cells thrive on iron. Mainstream tobacco smoke is estimated to contain as much as 0.1 percent of the metal contaminant; that is, 60,000 picograms of iron per cigarette smoked. Thus a one-pack/day smoker could inhale over one million picograms iron/day. In a number of reports, alveolar macrophages of smokers have been found to be brimming with iron—in many cases, in amounts sufficient to prevent the alveolar macrophages from killing cancer cells and pathogenic microbes.

Workplace: When working with asbestos, iron ore, steel, or scrubbing rust off metal objects such as automobiles, patio furniture, etc., inhalation of iron oxide dust can be inhibited by wearing a mask.

Cookware: Avoid iron skillets, stainless steel aluminum, enamelware, and foods cooked on a grill, especially at restaurants.

Minute filings of metal are released from these types of cookware and get into the food. When you eat these foods you ingest the filings, thus contributing to your iron intake.

Humans have specific enzymes that affect how much medication gets into circulation. One or more of the chemicals, possibly flavonoids, in grapefruit juice alter the activity of these enzymes, allowing for larger amounts of certain drugs to reach the bloodstream, resulting in increased activity and possibly toxicity, especially with drugs that have a narrow therapeutic index. In this type of medication even a moderate increase in blood levels could result in increased and even fatal arrhythmias.

WARNING!!!

Grapefruit juice can cause serious and dangerous side effects, including fatalities, when taken with certain medications. Something in the fruit causes drug potency to be increased up to twelve fold.

Medications that may be affected by grapefruit juice include calcium channel blockers used for high blood pressure and angina (chest pain), statin drugs used to lower cholesterol, some antihistamines, erythromycin, and some antifungals. Also affected are medications used to treat gastrointestinal disorders, tranquilizers, and protease inhibitors.

Anyone taking this type of medication can check with his or her pharmacist or physician for information about drug interaction.

Bacteria: Raw shellfish such as oysters can be infected with a bacteria called Vibrio vulnificus, which can be deadly to a person with high iron. Yersinia is another bacteria known to be harmful to those with elevated tissue iron.

Multivitamins: Many of us need the added benefit of a daily supplement, but those with an iron loading disorder do not need the extra iron contained in most supplements. These individuals should look for vitamins that contain no iron and provide the complete B-complex, and at least 400 IU of vitamin E, which is a good antioxidant. There are no known multivitamin supplements without C. Vitamin C enhances absorption of all nutrients and thus is included in an effort to assure optimum absorption. Females are often told to take supplemental calcium. Even though calcium is a known inhibitor of iron, calcium is best taken at bedtime because not only does it inhibit the absorption of iron, but many other essential nutrients and some medications.

Look for multivitamins without iron and low amounts of vitamin C. Spectravite™ for seniors, a CVS Drugs product, is a good choice. This product is especially important for older people with iron loading conditions, but also because elderly citizens are prone to anemia of chronic disease, and are often prescribed iron pills mistakenly.

Sugar: Consumed in large quantities such as found in soft drinks, sugar adds stress on the kidneys, liver, and pancreas. Moreover, sugar feeds bacteria and contributes to the development of plaques, which destroy gum tissue and eventually lead to tooth loss. Sugar also affects blood glucose levels, causing frequent surges of insulin to be released. Heavy consumption of sugar can contribute to weight gain, pancreatic exhaustion, and type 2 diabetes. Refined sugar is in many processed foods and even medicines. Though sugar substitutes have fewer calories than other types of sweeteners, many people will overindulge in these beverages not realizing that low-calorie eventually adds up.

WARNING!!!

DO NOT EAT RAW SHELLFISH *and*

TAKE CARE WALKING ON THE BEACH

Some shellfish contain a bacteria called Vibrio vulnificus, which can be fatal to a person with high iron levels

Water: Being properly hydrated, especially during therapeutic removal of blood, will reduce the amount of time it takes to remove a unit of blood. Also, a person will not run the risk of becoming dehydrated following therapy. Water also helps digest food and move waste through the intestine; this is especially important when consuming fiber, where added water is needed for this reason. People who drink well water that contains high levels of iron are getting about 1 milligram of iron per gallon of water. Wells can be tested for iron content and individuals who are in therapy, especially during the initial de-ironing period, might consider drinking distilled bottled water.

Fad diets: Fat-free diets are typically high in sugar and sodium. Zero-carbohydrate or low-carbohydrate diets are higher in fats and sodium. Medically recommended diets, such as the American

Heart Association Diet and American Diabetes Diet, are best; these diets can be adjusted to reduce iron content and absorption.

Exercise: We need exercise to strengthen bones and to keep from losing muscle tone, which includes the heart. As little as twenty minutes a day of regular activity can provide benefit. Strenuous exercise can result in blood loss, but most of us are not marathon runners. For people over fifty, especially those who have hormonal imbalances where metabolism has slowed, regular exercise is most important. Sticking with a routine is the most difficult part of an exercise program. Sometimes we allow busy schedules, boredom, fatigue, or weather conditions to thwart our plans, and before we realize it, exercise is no longer a part of our daily routine.

One good way to stick with a program is to find an exercise that is fun, such as dancing to your favorite music. Music offers a distraction from the tedium and helps the time pass quickly. Incorporating exercise into a daily routine in increments is a very good way to assure adequate activity is achieved. Modify the day's activities so that additional exertion takes place. For example, park a distance from the store entrance or your place of work so that you walk a few extra paces. Be conscious of your behavior and opportunities to move.

Aspirin: One baby aspirin taken daily can contribute to blood loss. Though the amount of loss is small, over the years the loss has an effect.

Blood donation (see facing page): An adult male can reduce his risk of heart attack by 50 percent with one blood donation a year. One blood donation contains about 250 milligrams of iron and is approximately equivalent to a year's blood loss experienced by menstruating females. It is not surprising that females with hemochromatosis do not begin to manifest heart trouble until 15 to 20 years after their periods have stopped.

Other tips that can be helpful:
- Arrange for treatment before you travel.
- Use ibuprofen as a pain reliever, not acetaminophen, which is harder on the liver. Be aware: Some ibuprofen products are coated with iron oxide; the amount is minimal but it is still iron.
- If you travel overseas get vaccinated for both hepatitis A and B.

Comparing Blood Donors

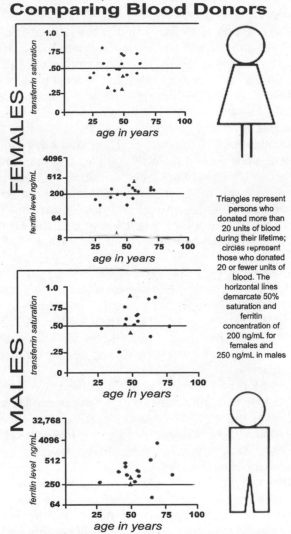

Triangles represent persons who donated more than 20 units of blood during their lifetime; circles represent those who donated 20 or fewer units of blood. The horizontal lines demarcate 50% saturation and ferritin concentration of 200 ng/mL for females and 250 ng/mL in males

Adapted with permission 2000 *American College of Physicians American Society of Internal Medicine*: The Effect of HFE Genotypes on Measurements of Iron Overload in Patients attending a Health Appraisal Clinic: E. Beutler, V. Felitti, T. Gelbart, N.Ho

- Get vaccinated for hepatitis A regardless.
- Don't become complacent about treatment.
- Be prepared; when you move to a new area, become familiar with local facilities before you have need for them.

These final two points are illustrated in the story of Eric.

Twenty-year-old Eric did not want to donate blood. He was too busy getting ready to go off to college and just didn't want to take the time to drive across town to the local blood center. Diagnosed with an iron loading disorder at the age of sixteen, and successfully de-ironed, Eric felt the situation was under control. He had plenty of time to go give blood.

Joint pain had been his biggest problem, and Advil took care of that, so the donation could wait a while, after all, how fast could iron accumulate? His family doctor had just tested his iron levels. Ferritin was not too high, 60-something, he remembers; and saturation percentage, he couldn't quite recall, but it was high, according to the doctor. Maybe that was the 60-something number. *Next time*, he thought, *I'd better write those numbers down somewhere.*

Weeks became months; his concerned mother asked about his blood donation schedule. Eric agreed it would be taken care of within the week. School was hypnotic, new friends, good grades, and great professors kept Eric distracted from his responsibility to give blood. Realizing it was Friday, and he had agreed to donate blood within the week, he rushed out the door to take care of the matter.

There was no blood donation center in the town where he went to school, so he would have to go to the one in his hometown, which was almost a two-hour drive. Fridays were the only days he could leave school because of classes, so Eric headed for the blood center back home. When he arrived, it was closed. *Oh well, next time*, thought Eric.

During the next few months Eric noticed his hair was thinning. Joint pain seemed a bit worse, and now he was having headaches, something he rarely got. Another problem he was reluctant to mention was sex-related. Eric noticed his desire for sex was waning. Though he was not thinking about marriage, he worried about the lack of feeling desire, which should be normal for his age.

226

After a lengthy discussion about these symptoms with a friend, Eric felt better; he realized his symptoms were probably related to his iron metabolism condition. He decided he would be more compliant with therapy, give up cola drinks and take some supplements. That Friday he gave blood. The following week he got sick. Chills, sweating, fever, headache, dizziness, and muscle aches caused Eric to miss class for the first time that semester.

He had e-mailed his mom that he was sick and told her the symptoms. She e-mailed back for him to get to the health center immediately. Worried about the potentially lethal combination of virus or bacteria and excess iron, she called Eric. He sounded somewhat better, but still she was concerned. Though there are no studies to support death by viral or bacterial infection except in the cases of yersinia and vibrio, she didn't want her son to take any chances.

It was 4:00 P.M. Eric had agreed to check out the school health center, buy a thermometer, and to call home by 10:00 A.M. the next morning. Forgetting that Eric was to call her the next morning, she called her son's room at 7 P.M. and got the answering machine. Hopeful that he was just sleeping, she left a message. The next morning her son's usual update and hello was not among her e-mail. At 7:00 A.M. she called her son's room. Again, she got the answering machine.

Reality hit, and panic replaced reason. She realized she did not know the main number of the campus, her son's room number, the name of the hospital, or the health center on campus. The only thing she could remember about Eric's girlfriend, Julie-something, was that she had long brown hair. She didn't know how to reach Eric's father, who was remarried and living elsewhere.

She dialed one more time and, to her relief, she heard the familiar, albeit sleepy voice of her twenty-year-old son through the receiver. He had gone to the pharmacy to buy a thermometer to see if he still had a fever. He had taken an over-the-counter cold and sinus medication and had slept deeply, his fever finally breaking.

The two talked about the lethal combination of iron and certain microorganisms, and about how fortunate it was that Eric had just removed 250 milligrams of iron with the recent blood donation. They discussed writing down contact numbers, knowing the local emergency health services, and being prepared when an emergency arises. Eric visited the college campus health center to learn that though they don't provide therapeutic phlebotomy, they will provide immunization for hepatitis A and B, and meningitis.

Since Eric had let his hepatitis A booster lapse, he was able to take advantage of the college health services for a very small charge. He then went to the emergency room and met with the director of Emergency Services and wrote out a contact list for the floor counselor, his mom, dad, and one close friend. He contacted Iron Disorders Institute Patient Services and asked them to send the ER physician and the hospital health center a letter about his condition. IDI sent a Patient Relocation Information Package to both the ER physician and the health center.

When a person waits until the crisis hits, panic will likely cause that person to do something that will be regrettable later on. Eric's mom is an educated woman. She has an important and demanding job, two factors that kept her from getting details that would have lessened her anxiety over of this experience.

Creating Your Personal Diet Plan
Good diet plans are ones that provide balance without disrupting a person's routine by completely eliminating favorite foods. Someone with an iron loading condition such as hemochromatosis will want to choose food combinations that impede iron reaccumulation, and cut back on foods that are high in meat-based iron. Like counting calories, a person will eventually learn which foods will help or hinder success of the plan.

- Make a list of the foods you like best. Create a sample breakfast, lunch, and dinner; include snacks. Examine your sample meals for the amount of meat-based iron versus plant-based iron. Adjust where you can to reduce the amount of meat-based iron. Incorporate into your diet food items that impede absorption, such as strong coffee, tea, and high-phytate foods. Absorption of meat-based iron cannot be impaired, therefore cutting back on meat consumption is key to reducing iron intake. There are several ways to cut back without forfeiting a favorite food such as red meat:

- reduce the number of red meat portions consumed weekly
- choose poultry, lean cuts of meat, and fish as alternatives to red meat
- eat smaller portions or
- eat combinations such as 1/2 portion of beef with 1/2 portion of chicken
- substitute ground turkey, chicken, or lean pork for beef in chili, meatloaf, and casserole dishes

Sample Menu

Breakfast
  Whole grain cereal, half a banana, skim milk, and coffee or tea
  Wheat bran and oatmeal cereals contain higher amounts of phytates than rice or corn cereals
Midmorning snack
  Tomato juice (or V8) and 1 oz. hard cheese
Lunch
  Chicken salad plate with rye krisps, cottage cheese and peaches, iced coffee or tea
Afternoon snack
  Apple wedge with peanut butter
Dinner
  Turkey chili served with crusty garlic toast and fresh green salad, tea or coffee

Turkey Chili

Sauté $^1/_2$ cup finely diced onion in 2 T olive oil
Add 2 pounds ground turkey; continue to cook until meat is done
Add 2 Tablespoons finely chopped parsley
Add 1 #28-oz. can diced or crushed tomatoes
Simmer $^1/_2$ hour until tomatoes are tender
Add: 1 10-oz. can of tomato sauce
$^1/_2$ cup Heinz catsup
Salt and red pepper to taste
Simmer 1 hour
Drain and rinse 1 #15-oz. can of dark red kidney beans

Add to chili mixture, bring back to boil
Cut off heat, let stand 15 minutes before serving

Yields 4 servings
From *Cooking with Iron*

TURKEY CHILI		*per serving* FOOD VALUES				
IRON MILLIGRAMS	FAT GRAMS	CARBOS GRAMS	FIBER GRAMS	PROTEIN	CALORIES	
heme ■ nonheme	animal ■ plant					
.9 5.4	13.2 .5	29.4	2	46.2	424	

This sample meal is designed to be low in heme iron (1 percent is meat-based), contain foods that will impede non-heme iron (phytates and dairy), <100milligrams of vitamin C with entrées, and is low-fat (only 13 grams of animal fat). Use the food values charts to create your own weekly meal plan.

Food Values Chart

Food and serving size	Iron	Vit.C	fat	fiber
iron and C expressed in milligrams--fat and fiber expressed in grams				
Beverages				
Beer, 12 fl. oz.	0.11	0	0	-
Coffee, brewed, 6 fl. oz.	0.72	0	0	-
Cola, 12 fl. oz.	0.13	0	0.1	-
Lemonade, from frozen concentrate, 6 fl. oz.	0.41	10	0.1	-
Lemon-lime soda, 12 fl. oz.	0.25	0	0	-
Milk, low-fat, 1% butterfat, 8 fl. oz.	0.12	2	2.6	-
Milk, nonfat, 8 fl. oz.	0.10	2	0.4	-
Milk, whole, 3.7% butterfat, 8 fl. oz.	0.12	4	8.9	-
Tea, black, brewed 3 min, 6 fl. oz.	0.04	0	0	-
Water (tap water), 8 fl. oz.	0.01	0	0	-
Wine, red table wine, 3.5 fl. oz.	0.44	0	0	
Wine, white table wine, 3.5 fl. oz.	0.33	0	0	-
Candy				
Almond Joy, Peter Paul, 1 oz.	0.44	0	2.3	1
Snickers 2-oz.	0.35	0	14	1
Caramels, 1 oz.	0.4	0	2.9	-
Chocolate, bittersweet, 1 oz.	1.4	0	11.3	-
Chocolate, semisweet, Bakers, 1/4 cup	1.11	0	11.8	-

Food Values Chart

Food and serving size	Iron	Vit.C	fat	fiber
Iron and C expressed in milligrams--fat and fiber expressed in grams				
Milk chocolate, 1oz.	0.3	0	9.2	-
Peanut butter cups, Reese's, 2 pieces (1.8 oz.)	0.56	-	16.7	-
Corn Chex, Ralston Purina, I cup	1.8	15	0.2	0
Cornflakes, Kellogg's, 1 1/4 cups	1.8	15	0.1	0
Cracklin' bran, Kellogg's, 1/3 cup	1.8	15	4.1	6
Complete Oat Bran, Kellogg's	7.5	0	0	4
Fruit & fiber, Post, with dates, raisins, walnuts, 1/2 cup	4.44	0	0.8	5
Granola, Nature Valley, 1 bar	0.95	-	4.9	3
Granola, Post Hearty Granola, 1/4 cup	4.44	0	4.1	0
Nutri-grain, Kellogg's, wheat, 3 /4 cup	0.8	15	0.3	4
Product 19,	18.0	60	0.2	-
Quaker 100% Natural, 1/4 cup	0.85	-	5.6	-
Raisin bran, Kellogg's, 2/3 cup	4.5	-	0.7	5
Rice Krispies, Kellogg's, 1 cup	1.8	15	0.2	-
Shredded wheat 1oz.	1.2	-	0.6	-
Special K, Kellogg's, 11/3cups	4.5	15	0.1	

Food Values Chart

Food and serving size	Iron	Vit.C	fat	fiber
iron and C expressed in milligrams--fat and fiber expressed in grams				
Total, General Mills Mills, 1 cup	18.0	0	0.6	2.4
Wheaties, General Mills, 1 cup	4.45	15	0.5	-
Other breakfast cereals: 1 cup cooked/plain				
Oatmeal	1.6	0	2.4	2.1
Cream of Wheat	10.3	0	0.7	-
Grits	1.5	0	-	0.6
Cheese and Cheese Products				
Cheddar, 1 oz.	0.19	0	9.4	0
Cottage cheese, 2% butterfat, 1 cup	0.36	0	4.4	0
Swiss, 1 oz.	0.05	0	7.1	0
Desserts				
Brownie, with nuts, homemade, 2 x2 piece	0.4	0	6.3	-
Cake, angel food, 1 piece	0.51	0	0.1	-
Cake, carrot, from Duncan Hines Deluxe Mix	0.62	-	4.0	-
Cake, cheesecake, 1/12 serving	0.41	4	16.3	-
Cake, devil's food, from mix, 1/12	0.70	0	11.3	-
Cake, gingerbread, from mix, 1/9 cake	1.0	0	4.3	-
Cake, white, from Mix, 1/12 cake	0.50	0	10.2	-
Cookie, chocolate chip, 1 3"	0.2	-	3	-
Cookie, oatmeal raisin, 1 3"	0.4	-	2.2	0.1

Food Values Chart

Food and serving size	Iron	Vit.C	fat	fiber
iron and C expressed in milligrams--fat and fiber expressed in grams					
Ice cream, vanilla, regular (10% butterfat), 1 cup	0.12	1	14.3	0
Pie, apple, homemade, 1/8	1.06	0	11.9	-
Pie, pumpkin, homemade, 1/8	0.60	0	12.8	-
Sherbet, orange, 1cup	0.31	4	3.8	0
Eggs and Egg Dishes				
Egg, boiled, hard or soft, I large	1.04	0	5.6	0
Popular Fast Foods				
Burger King Whopper	4.88	14	41.0	-
Kentucky Fried Chicken, original recipe, breast	0.63	-	13.7	-
Kentucky Fried Chicken, original recipe, drumstick	0.60	-	8.8	-
McDonald's Big Mac	4.9	3	35.0	-
McDonald's Chicken McNuggets, 1 serving	1.25	2	21.3	-
McDonald's Egg McMuffin	2.93		15.8	-
McDonald's french fries, 1 regular serving	0.61	13	11.5	-
McDonald's hamburger	2.85	2	11.3	-
Wendy's chicken broiled	2.7	1	19.0	-
Wendy's chili	3.2	0	11.0	2.6

Food Values Chart

Food and serving size	Iron	Vit.C	fat	fiber
iron and C expressed in milligrams--fat and fiber expressed in grams				
Pizza, cheese, 1 slice	1.61	2	8.6	-
Taco, 1	1.15	1	10.4	1.9
Fish, Shellfish,and Crustacea				
WARNING: DO NOT EAT RAW SHELLFISH				
Clams 4 large, 9 small	11.88	-	0.8	
Cod, baked or broiled, 3 oz.	0.41	1	0.7	0
Crab, Alaskan King, 3 oz.	0.5	-	0.5	0
Fish sticks, frozen, 1 stick	0.21	-	3.4	0
Haddock, baked or broiled, 3 oz.	1.14	-	0.8	0
Halibut, baked or broiled, 3 oz.	0.91	-	2.5	0
Lobster, boiled, 3 oz	0.33	-	0.5	0
Oysters, 6 medium	5.63	-	2.1	0
Salmon, pink, canned with bone, 3 oz.	0.72	0	5.1	0
Scallops, raw, 3 oz. 6 large or 14 small	0.25	-	0.6	0
Shrimp, boiled, 3 oz. (15 large)	2.62	-	0.9	0
Swordfish, baked or broiled, 3 oz.	0.88	1	4.4	0
Tuna, canned in oil, light, 3 oz.	1.18	-	7.0	0
Tuna, canned in oil, white, 3 oz.	0.56		6.9	0
Tuna, canned in spring water, light, 3 oz.	2.72		0.4	0

Food Values Chart

Food and serving size	Iron	Vit.C	fat	fiber

iron and C expressed in milligrams--fat and fiber expressed in grams

Fruit and Vegetable juices

Food and serving size	Iron	Vit.C	fat	fiber
Apple juice, canned or bottled, 8 fl. oz.	0.92	2	0.3	0
Grapefruit juice, canned, 8 fl. oz.	0.50	72	0.2	0

WARNING: Grapefruit juice can cause drug reactions with certain medicines

Food and serving size	Iron	Vit.C	fat	fiber
Orange juice, from frozen concentrate, 8 fl. oz.	0.24	97	0.1	0
Tomato juice 6 fl. oz	1.06	33	0.1	0
V-8, vegetable cocktail, 6 fl.oz	1.00	37	0.1	-

Fruits

Food and serving size	Iron	Vit.C	fat	fiber
Apple, with skin, 1 medium	1.06	8	0.25	1.1
Cantaloupe, pieces, 1 cup	0.34	68	0.4	1.0
Grapefuit, pink or red, 1/2 medium	0.15	47	0.1	0.2

WARNING: Grapefruit is not recommended when taking some high blood pressure medicines

Food and serving size	Iron	Vit.C	fat	fiber
Grapes, seedless 1 cup	0.27	4	0.3	0.7
kiwi fruit (1)	0.3	74.5	0.3	0.8
Orange, navel, 1 medium	0.13	69.7	0.1	0.6
Peach, fresh, 1 medium	0.47	3	0.1	0.6
Pear, fresh, 1 medium	0.41	7	0.7	2.2
Pineapple, fresh 1 cup	0.6	24	0.3	8.4

Food Values Chart

Food and serving size	Iron	Vit.C	fat	fiber
iron and C expressed in milligrams--fat and fiber expressed in grams				
Prunes, dried, 10 prunes	2.08	3	0.4	6.0
Raisins, seedless, 1/3 cup	2.08	3	0.5	4.0
Strawberries, fresh, 1 cup	0.57	85	0.6	3.4
Watermelon, pieces, 1 cup	0.28	15	0.7	2.8
Grain Products				
Bagel	1.46	0	1.4	1.6
Corn bread, from 2 x2 piece	0.80	0	5.8	3.4
French bread, 1 4" slice	0.92	-	1.1	-
Pita bread, 1 "pocket"	0.92	0	0.6	-
Pumpernickel bread, 1 slice	0.88	0	0.8	4.0
Raisin bread, 1slice whole wheat	0.78	0	1.0	6.5
Rye bread, 1 slice	0.68	0	0.9	3.4
Spaghetti, enriched, cooked,1 cup	2.25	0	0.7	2.4
White bread, 1 slice	0.68	0	0.9	0.4
Whole wheat bread, 1 slice	0.84	0	1.0	1.4

Food Values Chart

Food and serving size	Iron	Vit.C	fat	fiber
Meats and Poultry				
Beef, ground extra lean, pan-fried, 3.5 oz.	2.36	0	16.4	0
Beef, ground, regular, pan-fried 3.5 oz.	2.45	0	22.6	0
Beef, liver, pan-fried, 16 oz.	6.28	23	8.0	0
Beef, round, top separable lean and fat broiled, 3.5 oz.	2.81	0	8.8	0
Beef, short-loin, T-bone steak, lean and fat broiled, 3.5 oz. separable	2.54	0	24.6	0
Chicken, dark meat without skin, roast, 3.5 oz.	1.33	0	9.7	0
Chicken, light meat without skin, roast, 3.5 oz.	1.14	0	10.9	0
Lamb, leg, roast 3 oz.	1.40	0	16.1	0
Pork, center loin, pan-fried, 3.5 oz.	0.84	0	30.5	0
Pork, cured bacon, broiled or pan-fried, 3 medium pieces	0.31	6	9.4	0
Turkey, light meat 3.5 oz.	1.09	0	6.6	0
Turkey, dark meat 3.5 oz.	1.29	0	6.7	0

Food Values Chart

Food and serving size	Iron	Vit.C	fat	fiber
iron and C expressed in milligrams—fat and fiber expressed in grams				

Nuts and Seeds 1oz=1/4 cup

Almonds, toasted, 1 oz.	1.40	0	14.4	2.4
Cashews, dry-roasted ' I oz.	1.70	0	13.2	1.1
Coconut, dried, sweetened, 1 cup	1.33	0	23.8	3.4
Peanut butter, JIF 1 tablespoon	0.30	0	8.2	1.9
Peanuts, dry-roasted, 1 oz.	0.63	0	13.9	2.3
Sunflower seeds, dry-roasted, 1 oz.	1.1	0	14.1	0.5
Walnuts, black, dried, 1 oz.	0.87	-	16.1	1.1

Vegetables

Asparagus, boiled, 6 spears	0.59	18	0.3	1.7
Avocado, raw, California, 1 med.	2.04	14	30.0	8.5
Beans, baked, 1/2 cup.	3.00	5	4.0	7.0
Broccoli, boiled, 1/2 cup	0.89	49	0.2	2.3
Cabbage, green, boiled, 1/2cup	0.29	18	0.1	1.5
Carrot, raw, 1 medium	0.36	7	0.1	2.2
Cauliflower, boiled, 1/2 cup	0.26	34	0.1	1.7
Celery, raw, 1 stalk	0.19	3	0.1	0.7
Chickpeas (garbanzo beans), canned, 1 cup	3.23	9	2.7	1.0
Corn, yellow, boiled, 1/2cup	0.50	5	1.1	2.3

Food Values Chart

Food and serving size	Iron	Vit.C	fat	fiber
iron and C expressed in milligrams--fat and fiber expressed in grams				
Green beans (snap beans), boiled, 1/2 cup	0.79	6	0.2	2.0
Kidney beans, red, boiled, 1 cup	5.20	2	0.9	13.1
Lima beans, boiled,1 cup	4.36	0	0.7	6.6
Mushrooms, raw, 1/2 cup sliced	0.43	1	0.2	1.4
Onions, boiled, 1/2 1/2 cup	0.21	6	0.2	1.4
Peas, green, boiled, 1/2 cup	1.24	11	0.2	3.5
Peppers, sweet, raw, 1/2 cup	0.63	64	0.2	1.0
Potato, baked with skin, 1 med	1.00	26	0.2	2.4
Rice, brown, cooked,1 cup	1.00	0	1.2	3.5
Rice, white, enriched, cooked, 1 cup	1.80	0	0.2	1.0
Spinach, boiled, 1/2 cup	3.21	9	0.1	2.2
Sweet potato, baked, 1 med	0.52	28	0.1	3.4
Tomato, red, raw,1 medium	0.59	22	0.3	0.8

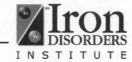

PART SEVEN

Support Across the USA and
Around the World

When people are first diagnosed with hemochromatosis, they experience an immediate heightened concern about the future of their health. This reality sensitizes them to their own mortality, and how hemochromatosis might affect their families. Unanswered questions about therapy, missed diagnoses, efforts to bring about awareness, research, and physician education can be overwhelming.

Reason can sometimes give way to emotion, especially when these individuals are met with disinterest about hemochromatosis from their physicians. People can feel they are waging war against an unseen adversary and that they are completely alone. The idea of being alone can frighten anyone, especially when a person's health is concerned. We all want to believe that no matter how our health is today, that there are groups of people working on behalf of such important matters as our health and well-being for the future and that support is available.

This section is about support. It provides highlights of U.S. iron experts, private organizations, public health agencies, and research under way specific to iron. These ongoing efforts throughout the USA, and around the world, can benefit anyone diagnosed with hemochromatosis, as well as numerous others who have not as yet been diagnosed.

29

About the Iron Disorders Institute (IDI)

People often ask us how Iron Disorders Institute (IDI) began. IDI got its beginnings much like our alliances around the world. Iron Disorders Institute was founded because of frustrations with out-dated ideas, attitudes of physicians who would not take hemochromatosis seriously, and because iron and its imbalances seemed to be at the core of so many health problems. Each of us at IDI has had a personal experience with iron imbalance disorders; most of us have hemochromatosis or we are directly caring for someone who has hemochromatosis. Founders of the organization believe that iron and its potential for harm is far too great for a single individual to address. It will take many working together cooperatively before this health issue moves forward.

Iron Disorders Institute is not affiliated with any other organization except through its alliances. IDI is not a membership-based organization; at present, it would be appropriate to say the organization is an educational resource center. Iron Disorders Institute produces educational materials, hosts scientific and patient conferences, and conducts workshops for nurse practitioners and technical staff such as phlebotomists. IDI is in the process of collecting camera-ready film footage that can be used for public service announcements and to produce documentaries about hemochromatosis. Iron Disorders Institute seeks advice from its Scientific Advisory Board, organizes the materials, and publishes booklets, pamphlets, and a quarterly magazine based on the advice of this board.

Iron Disorders Institute's Mission Statement: to reduce pain, suffering, and unnecessary death due to disorders of iron such as anemia of chronic disease, iron loading anemia, iron deficiency anemia, porphyria cutanea tarda, African siderosis, non-HFE–related iron overload, and hereditary hemochromatosis.

The fundamental premise on which Iron Disorders Institute is based includes that iron's influence and imbalances are the underlying cause of many health problems we face today, and may face in the future.

Strategies:

- Bring about consensus among U.S. scientists by providing for scientific conferences expressly for scientists and hosted by our Scientific Advisory Board. Matters such as USA laboratory values, diagnostic approaches, therapy, and maintenance guidelines for disorders of iron are key issues currently under consideration.

- Publish quality materials reviewed by experts so that these materials can serve to educate both the medical community and the public about disorders of iron such as hemochromatosis.

- Educate physicians about HHC, directly and indirectly with the help of HHC patients, the U.S. Centers for Disease Control, and Prevention and Scientific Conferences (One HHC patient might lead to the diagnosis of an entire family, but one physician who knows how to identify HHC can diagnose an entire community.)

- Work to bring important resources to "a common ground" to lessen the duplication of efforts, and to expedite matters of importance, such as research and policy. The flower illustrates how these resources interact: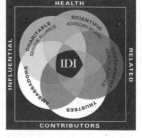

IDI Board of Trustees: The governing body of the organization assures that IDI fulfills its mission. Dr. Elliott Sigal, Vice President Applied Genomics; Richard Harrington, President & CEO The Harrington Group; Dr J. T. Ford, Past President of Independent Colleges of Georgia; Laura Main, Cheryl Garrison, Chris Kieffer, and Randy S. Alexander,

Chairman, make up the current Board of Trustees.

Scientific Advisory Board Members: Experts in iron who provide that the organization's printed materials, conference, and workshop content are medically accurate and scientifically current. Members appear in alphabetical order (following the Chairman and Vice-Chairman):

Herbert L. Bonkovsky, M.D., Iron Disorders Institute chairman

Dr. Bonkovsky is professor in the Departments of Biochemistry & Molecular Pharmacology and Medicine of the University of Massachusetts Medical School. He is the Fellowship Director, Division of Digestive Disease and Nutrition, Director of the Liver, Pancreatic and Biliary Center, Director of the NIH-Funded Clinical Center for Study of Hepatitis C and Director of the Center for Study of Disorders of Iron and Porphyrin Metabolism.

Dr. Bonkovsky received his undergraduate degree from Earlham College, 1963. He has been the recipient of numerous awards and honors and memberships, such as the Merit Scholar, Emma and Frank Binz Memorial Scholar, Alpha Omega Alpha Member Borden Award for excellence in research as a medical student and the Mosby award for scholastic excellence.

Dr. Bonkovsky received his postdoctoral training at several prominent universities and centers including Duke University, Case Western Reserve, National Cancer Institute (NIH) Metabolism Branch. His medical residency was completed through Dartmouth Medical School and Yale University School of Medicine. Dr. Bonkovsky is recognized in the USA and Internationally as an expert in liver disorders, iron and porphrin metabolism. He has participated in numerous scientific conferences as a key presenter and has served on many consensus panels including the European Association for the Study of the Liver (EASL).

P. D. Phatak, M.D., Head of Hematology and Medical Oncology at Rochester General Hospital, Iron Disorders Institute Vice-Chairman

Dr. Phatak served as Medical Adviser to Mary Gooley Hemophilia Center, more recently renamed Hemo Center, Rochester. He has participated in numerous CDC focus group activities, most recently as a panel member for the CDC's Physician Education initiative. At Rochester General Hospital Dr. Phatak has been the lead investigator of a large population-based hemochromatosis screening program. He has written about the findings from this landmark study in annals of *Internal Medicine,* December 1998.

Prevalence of hereditary hemochromatosis in 16,031 primary-care patients Dr. Phatak is recognized in the USA and internationally as an expert in disorders of iron such as anemia and iron overload. He has participated in numerous scientific conferences as a key presenter and has served on many consensus panels including the European Association for the Study of the Liver (EASL). A new and groundbreaking study by Dr. Phatak and Dr. Ronald Sham, hematologist/oncologist at Rochester General Hospital, appeared in the December 1, 2000, issue of *Blood,* the official journal of the American Society of Hematology, Asymptomatic Hemochromatosis Subjects. Genotypic and Phenotypic Profiles attempts to correlate identified genetic variations with the patient's symptoms and degree of iron overload.

Ann Aust, Ph.D., Department of Chemistry and Biochemistry, Utah State
Dr. Aust is an expert in inhaled carcinogenic materials such as iron-containing asbestos and other particulants inherent in today's environment. Her work is cutting-edge and garnering attention by those interested in the relationship of iron and cancer, especially inhalation of tobacco smoke and lung disease.

John Beard, Ph.D., Professor of Nutrition, Pennsylvania State University
Dr. Beard has studied the effects of iron deficiency on cognitive and behavioral performance, thyroid metabolism, and thermoregulation for more than twenty years. His work includes investigating benefits of iron supplementation in youths, women of childbearing age and the elderly.

David Brandhagen, M.D., Department of Gastroenterology & Hepatology, Mayo Clinic
Dr. Brandhagen is a hepatologist specializing in diseases of the liver. In his practice, he treats more than two hundred hemochromatosis/ iron overload patients. His important clinical experience

in HHC is accented by numerous awards and honors, including the 1998 American Federation of Medical Research Award.

James Connor, Ph.D., Professor and Vice Chair, Department of Neuroscience & Anatomy, Director G.M. Leader Alzheimer's Disease Research Laboratory
Dr. Connor is recognized as an expert in the relationship between iron and neurodegenerative diseases. He is one of the first to make an association between hemochromatosis/iron overload and depression. His current work includes having identified an antibody to the divalent metal transporter DMT1 believed to play a significant role in iron absorption.

John Feder, Ph.D., Bristol-Meyers Squibb Pharmaceutical Research
Dr. Feder was a key participant on the HFE gene discovery team. Two prevalent mutations, C282Y and H63D, are now known to contribute to abnormal iron metabolism. His current work focuses on novel gene therapies, and he is an adviser to those pursuing genetic research.

Kris Kowdley, M.D., Department of Medicine, University of Washington, Seattle
Dr. Kowdley is a practicing hepatologist expert in liver transplantation. His interest in the role of hemochromatosis and the liver led him to organize a Hemochromatosis/ Iron Disorders Clinic in Seattle. He has written extensively about liver transplantation and is respected throughout the world for his work in this field.

John Longshore, Ph.D., Director of Molecular Diagnostics Greenwood Genetic Center
Dr. Longshore is an expert in molecular analysis. His findings in progress include possibility of higher prevalence of HFE mutation for hemochromatosis in the southern region on U.S. population and occurrence of C282Y in nonwhites.

Patrick MacPhail, M.D., Ph.D., Department of Medicine University of Witwatersrand

Dr. MacPhail is expert in African siderosis. His work includes research of relationship to iron overload and genetics in Africans.

David Meyers, M.D., M.P.H., Department of Medicine Division of Cardiovascular Disease, Kansas University Hospital
Dr. Meyers is an expert in cardiovascular disease. His more than two decades of work include writing Kansas Primary Care Physicians Preventive Health Guidelines. He provides scientific substantiation of a connection to reduced incidence of cardiac arrest and frequency of blood donation.

Jukka Salonen, M.D., Ph.D., MSc, P.H. Department of Medicine University of Kuopio
Dr. Salonen, a leading epidemiologist, conducted the first major study of incidence of cardiac attack in males relative to ferritin levels. His ongoing work includes incidence of cardiac attack in heterozygotes.

Barry Skikne, M.D., Kansas University Medical Center
Dr. Skikne is an expert in iron balance: excess or insufficiency. His more than twenty-five years in the field includes pioneer work on the serum transferrin receptor—one of the most sophisticated diagnostic revelations of the decade.

Nancy Olivieri, M.D., F.R.C.P (C), Hemoglobinapathy Program, The Hospital for Sick Children, Toronto, Canada
Dr. Olivieri is internationally known for her research and expertise of thalassemia. Over the past fifteen years, her work has included contributions to development of new approaches to therapy for those with thalassemia and sickle cell anemia.

Mark Princell. M.D., Director Emergency Room Services St. Francis Health System
Dr. Princell manages services for two major emergency room facilities. His knowledge of hemochromatosis/iron overload spans more than a decade. His current work in progress includes "Chest pain in the emergency room and possible hemochromatosis."

Eugene Weinberg, Ph.D., Professor of Microbiology, Indiana University
Dr. Weinberg is a leading expert in infectious disease and cancer. His work focuses on prevention of chronic disease by lowering iron levels by reducing intake of dietary iron and discontinuing contributive factors such as tobacco and alcohol use. His more than forty years work in the field of iron's relationship to cancer has earned him prestige and recognition worldwide. His recent paper in Emerging Infectious Diseases—a new CDC publication—is among over a hundred excellent articles he has written on the subject of iron and its carcinogenic and oxidant capabilities.

Emeritus Scientific Advisory Board Members
From time to time busy schedules and new opportunities arise for our SAB members. We appreciate the contributions of these esteemed scientists and understand when they cannot participate actively in IDI projects. In these situations we retire them to Emeritus status. In this way they continue to be acknowledged for their fine efforts and continue to receive certain privileges of active members. Among our Emeritus status SAB are:

Nancy Andrews, M.D., Ph.D., Department of Medicine, Howard Hughes Medical Institute at the Children's Hospital
Dr. Andrews was recently promoted to the position of Director of MD, MPh.D. Program at Harvard; she is also associate professor of hematology, oncology at Harvard Medical School and Associate Investigator for Howard Hughes Medical Institute. Her work continues to focus on red blood cell development, and iron metabolism. Dr. Andrews was instrumental in identifying a novel iron transport Nramp2, now known as DMT1. Her findings contribute greatly to a better understanding of iron transport and absorption.

Alan Buchanan, Ph.D., University of Arizona, is a medical ethicist. The focus of his work continues to include formulation of policy about the ethical, legal, moral, and social implications of genetic testing.

Charitable Health Alliances: National and international volun-tary health agencies that address various disease consequences of iron imbalances. Iron Disorders Institute educates a patient about iron imbalances, then refers them to the appropriate alliance expert or support group that can address a specific need. Charitable Health Alliances include: American Heart Association, Arthritis Foundation, American Liver Foundation, American Diabetes Association, Cooley's Anemia, Aplastic Anemia & MDS International Foundation, Hepatitis International, Mary Gooley Hemo Center, Restless Legs Syndrome, Genetics Alliance Support Group, State Genetic Counselors, International Alliances, and other health-related organizations.

Ambassadors: Are individuals who volunteer time to write, attend conferences, and distribute information about breaking news and events within their community.

Influential Health Related Contributors: This group includes medical universities, treatment centers, genetic laboratories, insurance industry, manufacturers of diagnostic aids and treatment equipment, publishers of health-related materials and radio/television/Internet health resources, and organizations such as the American Medical Association, the American Clinical Laboratories Association, and other well-established medical organizations.

Government Health Alliances include: USDHHS, Department of Health and Human Services, The Centers for Disease Control and Prevention, and The National Institutes of Health as well as other U.S. Government agencies such as the Veterans Administration, and the U.S. Department of Agriculture.

Iron Disorders Institute logo: The logo is comprised of two triangles, one red, the other one black representing iron excess
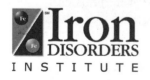
and insufficiency. Each one contains a round "Fe" object floating within the triangular shapes, which stand for the two atoms of iron carried by transferrin and the iron contained in ferritin. The triangles, when placed together, create a diagonal slash representing transferrin iron saturation percentage. As a whole, the logo symbolizes all things associated with iron balance.

Iron Disorders Institute mascot: Cartoon character CR Hume

is a ferret who is featured on promotional materials used to raise awareness about the importance of periodically checking iron levels. His name is a play on words; when said

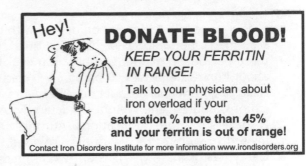

rapidly, CR Hume is meant to sound like "serum," and since he is a ferret, he represents serum ferritin. A contest to determine the meaning of CR's name was won by Arthur Callahan, Memphis, Tennessee.

Iron Disorders Institute's Products

Our products are reviewed by members of our Scientific Advisory Board and people at the U.S. Centers for Disease Control and Prevention. The professional look is due to the talents of Sandy Bowers of Bowers Creative, and Cheryl Garrison, IDI head of educational product development. Dave and Paul Malone of Elite Press provide offset printing; they trim, collate, and staple offset printed materials such as *idInsight*. Other products such as trifold pamphlets, booklets, posters, and transparencies are printed by Garrison Graphics. Pamphlets and booklets are collated and stapled by volunteers and by IDI staff Kay Owen and Donna Duncan.

Products available

Guide to: Diagnosing Hemochromatosis/Iron Overload: trifold pamphlet given free to patients upon request and customized to include local contact information for treatment centers such as HemoCenter Rochester, NY, and University of Massachusetts digestive disease, diagnostics and treatment center.

Guide to: Diagnosing Anemia trifold pamphlet given free to patients upon request and customized to include local contact information for treatment centers

Guide to: Treatment—Hemochromatosis/Iron Overload booklet that helps describe therapeutic phlebotomy and helpful hints during therapy.

Personal Health Profile

A four-page folder that can be helpful with record-keeping *idIn-sight* magazine, which as of 2001 first quarter issue includes *idIn-touch* newsletter: quarterly publication with five or more articles about iron-related issues. Topics are selected by Cheryl Garrison, Head of educational product development which includes publications, and Eugene Weinberg, Scientific Advisory Chair, Iron Disorders Institute Publications. Authors are scientific experts invited to write or review drafts provided by Dr. Weinberg or Cheryl Garrison. In years when two conferences (both patient and scientific) occur, such as even years (2000, 2002, 2004, etc.) IDI publishes only two issues of the magazine. Subscriber's renewal dates are adjusted to compensate.

Website www.irondisorders.org the IDI website was designed by Rusty Thompson, RainCloud Studios. He gave it its crisp, professional look and its user-friendly navigation. Content is provided by individuals in IDI educational product development, and reviewed by IDI Scientific Advisory Board Members and people selected from the IDI database.

About other organizations

Iron Disorders Institute cofounder Chris Kieffer contacted IOD, Hemochromatosis Foundation, and American Hemochromatosis Society to obtain permission to publish their mission statement, or website information. IOD and Hemochromatosis Foundation were not able to participate. Readers can visit their website: ironoverload.org or hemochromatosis.org and learn about these two pioneer organizations. Iron Disorders Institute commends everyone who has worked to bring awareness to this most important health issue known as hemochromatosis/iron overload disease.

American Hemochromatosis Society (AHS), established 1998, Del Ray Beach, Florida, Sandra Thomas, Founder. Mission Statement: The mission of the American Hemochromatosis Society (AHS) is to educate and support the victims of hereditary hemochromatosis and their families as well as educate the medical community on the latest research on HH. AHS's aim is to identify through genetic testing, the 35 million-plus Americans who unknowingly carrying the single or double gene mutation

252

for HH, which puts them at risk for loading excess iron.

AHS recognizes and envisions that it is possible now and in the future to prevent needless deaths, disability, organ damage, costly joint replacements and organ transplants caused by hereditary hemochromatosis/iron overload through:

- Routine/universal screening for HH of the American public
- DNA newborn screening for HH for all children in America
- Establishment of universal guidelines for diagnosis and treatment for HH in children and adults
- AHS projects, which involve patient, family, community, and governmental cooperation and support for screening and awareness include:
- "Children HHelping Children"™ Screening & Awareness Project for pediatric hereditary hemochromatosis
- "Seniors HHelping Seniors"™ Screening & Awareness Project for geriatric hereditary hemochromatosis
- "Hereditary Hemochromatosis Congressional Challenge"— DNA testing of all members of Congress
- "Hereditary Hemochromatosis Celebrity Challenge"—DNA testing of all celebrities, including those in the film and music industry.

30

International Alliances

Until the late 1970s there were no formally organized groups addressing the issue of hereditary hemochromatosis. Few people at that time had actually been diagnosed. Mayo Clinic, a United States health icon, had only thirteen confirmed cases of hemochromatosis by the mid-1960s. The condition was thought to be rare, an older male's disease.

As the world grew smaller through television, air travel, and people moved from city to city, or even to different countries, information about hemochromatosis began to emerge. Through the efforts of individuals like Marie Warder, Dr. Margit Krikker, and Roberta Crawford, gradually people with hemochromatosis had a source of information.

These pioneering women all shared a common goal, to raise awareness about hemochromatosis/iron overload. Marie Warder organized an international hemochromatosis network, which connected people worldwide on this issue. The Hemochromatosis Research Foundation in Albany, New York, founded by Dr. Margit Krikker, was the first U.S. organization to address hemochromatosis in America. Next was Iron Overload Diseases (IOD), Palm Beach, Florida, founded by Roberta Crawford.

For the next twenty years Warder, Krikker, and Crawford struggled to get the attention of physicians. They wrote countless letters, worked long hours, and gave generously of their time to speak anywhere in the world when asked to do so. Their stories are part of history and represent the beginnings of service to families with hemochromatosis/iron overload all over the world.

The Canadian Hemochromatosis Society, Richmond, British Columbia

Marie Warder figured out long before her physician that she was a carrier for hemochromatosis. Her husband, Tom, had been diagnosed in 1975, but not until their daughter Leigh was diagnosed in 1979 did Marie put it all together. Her family was living in Johannesburg, South Africa, at the time of Tom's diagnosis, but had moved to Canada by the time Leigh received her diagnosis. For Marie, it was the love of her family that inspired her and drove her to challenge theories that had become entrenched in the minds of many physicians. One theory she was determined to dispel was that premenopausal females do not accumulate iron. She looked at her 32-year-old daughter, who was living proof that menstruating females can indeed become overloaded with iron.

Marie wrote letters to newspapers and magazines but was met with indifference. As she encountered one family after another who seemed to find her regardless of where they lived in the world, Marie decided that an organization had to be established. In 1978 she started the Canadian Hemochromatosis Society. But it would be November 1982, after three years of struggle with financial setbacks and government red-tape, when the Canadian Hemochromatosis Society was finally incorporated with seven members.

By 1985 the CHS had over 450 members and an International Hemochromatosis Society Network beginning with South Africa, and stretching around the world to Great Britain, Australia, and France. Marie's family, Leigh, Tom, and Shaun helped her immeasurably to run the demanding network of societies. Marie appeared on television, in newspaper articles, and was written about in *Reader's Digest*. Her ardor was apparent when she challenged the Canadian Red Cross to take HHC blood, and persuaded Consumer and Corporate Affairs to change misleading "reduced iron" labels on food packages. Her drive to raise awareness, designating the month of May as "HHC Awareness Month" in Canada, resulted in the proper diagnosis of more than five hundred individuals. In June 1991, Marie was awarded the Canada Volunteer Award from the office of the health minister in recognition of her work. Her efforts are known in England,

Ireland, Holland, Belgium, France, Germany, Australia, the USA, and in South Africa.

The Bronze Killer, her book about the Warder family experience with hemochromatosis, is in its third printing. Now retired, Marie knows that her organization is in good hands. Charm Cottingham stepped in to continue a watchful eye over the organization that was started by Marie some twenty years earlier. Charm's husband died early as a result of hemochromatosis. His autopsy revealed massive upper gastrointestinal hemorrhage secondary to esophageal varices, which are varicose veins in the esophagus. He had hemochromatosis with cirrhosis, pancreatic atrophy, an enlarged heart, testicular atrophy and ascites, aortic valve damage, myocardial degeneration in the left ventricle, old renal infarcts, old right cerebral infarct, and old and recent splenic infarcts. He was only sixty-one. Charm continues to raise awareness on behalf of Canadians with hemochromatosis; she works with Marguie Nordman, Education and Development Director for CHS.

Today there are more than fifteen hemochromatosis organizations networked internationally. Now, early detection and treatment offer a unique opportunity to prevent chronic disease for millions of people worldwide. Marie Warder is to be credited with initiating events that resulted in this network of international organizations all devoted to alerting the world about this common hereditary condition. International Network of Societies are located Australia, United Kingdom, Dutch Netherlands, Italy, South Africa, Spain, Belgium, Brazil, Ireland, Israel, USA, the Ukraine, and New Zealand.

Pioneers in Preventive Medicine
Numerous health facilities throughout the USA are currently aware of how to diagnose hemochromatosis. Most of these health centers offer therapeutic phlebotomy and some are doing research about iron. The following centers, however, stand out as pioneers for their early recognition that detection of hemochromatosis presymptomatically offers an excellent opportunity to prevent chronic disease. One center in particular has the distinction of not only screening, diagnosing, and treating people with hemochromatosis, this center also provides its hos-

pital system with an endless supply of blood.

At Kaiser Permanente in San Diego, California, Director of Preventive Medicine Dr. Vincent Felitti has been recognized repeatedly for his efforts to identify and treat individuals with hemochromatosis. Dr. Felitti's interest in hemochromatosis began nearly forty years ago in the early 1960s when he was a medical student at the Johns Hopkins University School of Medicine. The disorder fascinated him, and over the years Dr. Felitti began to take an active role in how the disorder could benefit patients while having a positive impact on health care costs.

With the cooperation and support of Kaiser Permanente's Chief of Pathology Dr. Michael Bonin, and Dr. Ray Yip at the U.S. Centers for Disease Control and Prevention, Felitti established the first institutional screening program of its kind in the USA and possibly the first of its kind in the world.

Initially, the screening study involved 15,000 patients. Kaiser's efforts generated a report with findings that iron overload was as prevalent among Hispanics as it is among those of European descent. As a result of the benefits that resulted from this pilot study, Kaiser implemented the screening program as part of its routine policy to prevent chronic disease. Since 1995, under the guidance of Dr Vincent Felitti, Kaiser Permanente has screened more than 200,000 San Diego members for hereditary hemochromatosis.

Transferrin saturation is measured once in a lifetime on a random blood specimen for persons who are part of the Kaiser Health Plan in San Diego. If a TS level greater than 45 percent results, a fasting saturation is performed along with serum ferritin. If these are elevated, the genetic test is performed. When a patient is found to be homozygous, results of their genetic tests and educational materials and a videotape about hemochromatosis are mailed to the patient under the supervision of very bright and capable Naomi Howard, Research Coordinator. Educational materials developed by Dr. Felitti have been invaluable to the screening program. These materials and videotapes with accompanying booklets help educate patients about HHC prior to their return for follow-up consultation at which point the patient is started on an individualized treatment program. Patients are referred to Kaiser Blood Donor Center supervised by

Rose Hooper. ". . . a marvel at getting people through the initial fears and apprehensions associated with blood donation. Rose makes the donation process easy and effective," says Dr. Felitti.

Kaiser applied for and obtained its FDA variance for use of HHC blood for transfusion in October of 2000. Dr. Felitti points out that there is a great economic value to the use of this blood. Hooper reports that the number of pints of usable blood doubled each month solely as result of units obtained from HHC patients.

Another major screening study involving Kaiser and Dr. Felitti is about to conclude. Scripps Research Institute's Dr. Ernest Beutler, considered one of the "giants" in the study of iron-related disorders, and Dr. Felitti are working together on a large population-based study, funded by National Institutes of Diabetes and Digestive and Kidney Diseases (NIDDK). Drs. Beutler and Felitti are screening a total of 60,000 patients who registered for health appraisal and gave consent for DNA analysis. Extensive medical histories, laboratory tests, and DNA testing are performed on these participants, thus allowing for comparison of HHC patients with non-HHC patients. In this way, information about environmental impact and penetrance can be obtained en mass. Preliminary findings of the study reveal that screening for transferrin iron saturation and ferritin levels does not detect all homozygotes for the major hemochromatosis mutation, that not all homozygotes become symptomatic, and that heterozygotes for HFE have a lower prevalence for iron deficiency anemia.

Dr. Felitti was asked about major obstacles in physician education, to which he responded, "The biggest problem with physician awareness is that many physicians have an innate belief that HHC is rare. This belief starts in medical school and is self-perpetuating as a result of priorities. Physicians are too busy to read papers and articles unless the topics are of practical value for the kinds of patients they're seeing. Topics become interesting only when a physician is sensitized to an issue. Inundating physicians with literature about HHC will not likely have much of an effect on the ones who continue to think the disorder is rare. HHC has a real PR problem and it is incumbent upon us to increase physician awareness in ways that really work."

Dr. Felitti has found that videotapes are helpful in educating both physicians and patients. Recommended titles include:

Hemochromatosis, the Disease of Iron Overload (accompanied by a booklet)

Recommended for physicians only:

Hemochromatosis in Orthopedics and Rheumatology

Hemochromatosis in Cardiology

Hemochromatosis at Autopsy

Hemochromatosis Diagnosed Too Late

Dr. Felitti's tapes can be ordered directly through Naomi Howard (nxhoward@scal.kp.org) or from the Iron Disorders Institute Patient Services Manager Kay Owen (educational services@irondisorders.org).

Dr. Felitti is the first recipient of Iron Disorders Institute's "Making a Difference" award. This award is given to practicing clinicians in recognition of extraordinary efforts to detect, treat, and educate the public and medical community about hemochromatosis.

St. John's Health System, Springfield, Missouri, incorporates St. John's Regional Health Center and St. John's Physicians & Clinics and Visiting Nurse Association. The system serves a 32-county area in southwest Missouri and northwest Arkansas, including Springfield, a city of 150,000, delivering a full range of health care services.

Phlebotomy services are offered in collaboration with the Community Blood Center (CBC) of the Ozarks in Springfield, with other locations in Joplin and Springdale. The CBC offers phlebotomy for hemochromatosis at no charge to patients, and is experienced in management of hemochromatosis phlebotomy. Community Blood Center of the Ozarks applied for FDA variance in April 2000 to utilize hemochromatotic blood.

St. John's Health System became the home of a landmark HHC prevalence study, when in 1997, Dr. Alex Hover decided to take on a challenge made by colleague Dr. Jim Blaine. Blaine and Hover are prominently featured on the cover of the premiere issue of *idInsight,* Iron Disorders Institute's magazine. Dr. Blaine challenged Dr. Hover that hemochromatosis is common and underdiagnosed. Hover was skeptical, but took on that challenge and initiated screening 1,653 employees of St. John's Regional Staff. With the help of Donna Gloe, Ed Barber, the

Springfield/Greene County Health Department, Premier Health Plan, Advocates for a Healthy Community, and the U.S. Centers for Disease Control and Prevention, the study was under way. Of the 1,653 tested 13 met the case definition of HHC; 3 had elevated iron. Thus hemochromatosis was detected in ten persons prior to any symptoms or elevated iron levels. This scenario lends support for some type screening for HHC and the prevention of chronic disease.

The HemoCenter is an independent diagnostic treatment center that specializes in the care of blood-related genetic disorders, including hemophilia, von Willebrand's disease, and Hereditary Hemochromatosis (HH). The HemoCenter opened in 1959 as one of the first hemophilia treatment centers in the nation. The center has been treating hemochromatosis since 1991, and it is recognized for its expertise in comprehensive hemochromatosis care both locally and nationally. With more than 240 registered patients with iron overload, its aim is to raise awareness and increase the early diagnosis of hemochromatosis so patients can avoid or minimize serious complications. In addition to diagnosing and treating RFL, the center also promotes family screening and participates in numerous HH research studies.

Medical staff members include Dr. Pradyumna Phatak, chief of Medical Oncology and Hemotology at Rochester General Hospital (RGH) in Rochester, New York; Dr. Ronald Sham, hematologist/oncologist at RGH; and Dr. Peter Kouides, medical director of the HemoCenter and a hematologist at RGH specializing in von Willebrand's disease. Dr. Phatak was the principal investigator for the largest hemochromatosis screening study ever conducted. The Hemophilia Center coordinated the effort, which screened 16,000 patients through their primary-care doctors' offices. As a result, thirty-eight people were identified with RH and are being treated at the center. The screening study was published in the Annal of Internal Medicine in 1998.

A new and groundbreaking study by Drs. Phatak and Sham appeared in the December 1, 2000, issue of *Blood*, the official journal of the American Society of Hematology, Asymptomatic Hemochromatosis Subjects. Genotypic and Phenotypic Profiles attempts to correlate identified genetic variations with the patient's symptoms and degree of iron overload. Their current grant is titled Hemochromatosis: Genetic Prevalence and Penetrance.

Dr. Phatak serves on the Scientific Advisory Board of the Iron Disorders Institute.

Key people to contact at the HemoCenter:

Pradyumna D. Phatak, M.D.

Ronald L. Sham, M.D.

Peter A. Kouides, M.D.

Robert W. Fox, President/CEO

Lynn Kulzer, RN BSN, Director of Clinical Operations

Jennifer LaFranco, RN BSN, Nurse Coordinator

Carolynn Lecesse, RN BSN, Nurse

Linda Alongi, Consumer Advocacy Coordinator

Tricia Oppelt, CSW, Social Worker

Caroline Braggins, MBA, Research Manager

Susan Woehr, Director of P.R./Development

The Mary M. Gooley HemoCenter 1415 Portland Avenue, Suite 425 Rochester, NY 14621 Phone: 716 922-5700 Fax: 716 922-5775 www.hemocenter.org

University of Pennsylvania Hemochromatosis Clinic is one of the largest centers in the USA. Due to the leadership of Chris Friedrich, M.D., Ph.D., this facility offers genetic counseling and treatment for HHC.

At the Johns Hopkins Hospital, which has a long tradition of training geneticists who are interested in adult conditions, Friedrich first appreciated that hemochromatosis was, in fact, the most common genetic condition in the USA. He also learned that most geneticists were focused on pediatrics or obstetrics, and that no genetics clinics had major programs for hemochromatosis (although a handful of excellent programs did exist outside of genetics clinics).

Dr. Friedrich became convinced hemochromatosis should be thought of as an excellent condition for preventive medicine efforts. It is common, screening tests are widely available, an inexpensive treatment is available everywhere. Further, it had been demonstrated that early diagnosis, followed by regular treatment, could prevent almost all of the clinical problems associated with advanced disease. The genetic basis of the condition also made a genetics clinic the logical place to organize a program, since the people at highest risk of having the condition were relatives of those already diagnosed.

When Dr. Friedrich joined the faculty of the University of Pennsylvania in 1996, he made it a priority to develop a program for patients with hemochromatosis. The first step was to identify other specialists who were skilled at treating some of the common manifestations of hemochromatosis. This included hepatologists, rheumatologists, cardiologists, and endocrinologists. At about this time the gene responsible for most cases of hemochromatosis, now known as HFE, was identified, and two mutations were found to be associated with almost all cases. Working with our molecular diagnostics laboratory, Dr. Friedrich was soon able to add molecular testing and carrier testing to the biochemical testing already available from the hospital laboratory.

The next step was to make physicians and the community more aware of this condition. Dr. Friedrich worked with the major patient support groups for this condition, which began referring callers to the clinic for appointments. He also sent out letters to primary-care doctors in our region, gave talks to hospital and physician groups, and gave talks for the general public. He appeared on local television news, local and national radio shows, and was quoted in newspaper articles. His program was under way, and the goal to disease prevention was becoming a reality in his community.

In November 2000, Dr. Friedrich accepted a position at the University of Mississippi School of Medicine to launch a hemochromatosis program there. He plans to provide the same level of care to a population that does not yet have an organized program to prevent the complications caused by undiagnosed iron overload. Dr. Joseph Maher, an internist and geneticist at the VA Medical Center in Jackson, MS, has already developed the HFE genotyping test needed for this program, and sees veterans suspected of having hemochromatosis. Meanwhile, the University of Pennsylvania Clinic carries on with the program Dr. Friedrich implemented with the hope of preventing chronic disease.

Southern Iron Disorders Center, Birmingham, Alabama. Dr. James C. Barton began studying the absorption and metabolism of iron and nonferrous metals in 1975. When he started his center in 1990, his goal was to provide diagnosis, treatment, educational programs, and research participation opportunities for hemochromatosis and other iron-related disorders. He has evaluated and treated more than 600 persons with hemochromatosis and related disorders during the years his center has been in existence. Dr. Barton has authored over 140 nonabstract publications and has made numerous contributions to physician education about iron and hemochromatosis. Dr. Barton is coeditor with Corwin Q. Edwards, M.D., University of Utah, of the book *Hemochromatosis: Genetics, Pathogenesis, Diagnosis, and Treatment* (Cambridge University Press, 2000). This is the only current, comprehensive textbook written for medical doctors and other scientists on the subject of hereditary hemochromatosis and related areas of interest. An international team of 94 authors contributed to the book, which covers all aspects of pathophysiology, epidemiology, diagnosis and treatment of hemochromatosis.

Dr. Barton's research interests include absorption and metabolism of iron and nonferrous metals; lactoferrin metabolism; population and molecular genetics, clinical manifestations, and therapy of hemochromatosis and other forms of primary iron overload; Field Center and co-investigator site for current NIH hemochromatosis screening project (HEIRS).

Kris Kowdley, M.D., Department of Medicine University of Washington, Seattle Iron Disorders Institute Scientific Advisory Board Member

The Iron Overload Clinic at the University of Washington Medical Center was founded in 1998 by Dr. Kris V. Kowdley. Dr. Kowdley began his medical training at Mount Sinai School of Medicine in New York City. Upon completion in 1985, he moved to the West Coast to study at Oregon Health Sciences University where he completed his Internship and Residency. He completed a Fellowship in Gastroenterolgy and Hepatology at Tufts University School of Medicine. Besides his involvement with the Iron Overload Clinic, Dr. Kowdley is an attending physician at the University of Washington Medical Center and Associate Professor of Medicine.

Dr. Kowdley's interest in liver disease and iron overload began during his fellowship training in Boston. He participated in a study that examined hepatic iron deposition and hepatic iron concentration in various liver diseases. Since that time he has focused his interest on hereditary hemochromatosis. He attributes his interest in hemochromatosis to the support and mentorship provided by Dr. Marshall Kaplan in Boston and Dr. Tony Tavill in Cleveland. Over the last several years Dr. Kowdley has developed a keen interest in liver transplantation for hemochromatosis. He has published several articles in the area of liver transplantation for hemochromatosis, and also on the possible effect of hepatic iron overload on outcome after liver transplant in patients without hemochromatosis.

The Iron Overload Clinic at the University of Washington Medical Center specializes in the diagnosis and management of adults with iron overload disorders. Most patients seen in the clinic have hereditary hemochromatosis, the most common inherited condition in the United States. We also see patients with secondary iron overload, due to repeated blood transfusions, iron injections, or other causes.

The clinic is staffed by highly trained physicians from the UW School of Medicine's divisions of Gastroenterology and Hematology, as well as from Pathology and Medical Genetics. Our multidisciplinary services include genetic testing for the recently identified hemochromatosis gene, as well as genetic screening and counseling for family members of patients with hemochromatosis. We are also experienced in liver biopsy, one of the clinical tests often used to establish a diagnosis of iron overload disease.

Oklahoma Blood Institute
Apheresis is emerging as a good way to de-iron some patients. The same pretreatment qualifications as therapeutic phlebotomy apply, but according to Dr. James Smith of Oklahoma Blood Institute, apheresis is more efficient, albeit more expensive than phlebotomy.

Besides the Oklahoma Blood Institute (OBI), among the first centers in the USA to offer apheresis treatment specifically as a therapeutic option for individuals with iron overload is Reading Hospital System, Reading, Pennsylvania.

University of Alabama (UAB) Dr. Louis Heck became interested in hemochromatosis as a medical student when he saw a patient who had formerly been diagnosed with alcoholic hepatitis. Dr. Heck believed the patient when he said he had not consumed alcohol in more than twenty years. With the help of the staff physician, Dr. Heck witnessed his first diagnosis of hemochromatosis. This was more than twenty years ago. Dr. Heck specializes in rheumatoid arthritis. Dr. Heck gives lectures to first-year medical students about hemochromatosis and its rheumatic-like manifestations.

Mayo Clinic in Rochester, Minnesota, and Dr. Virgil Fairbanks offered some of the first information and treatment for hemochromatosis. Mayo continues to expand its services for patients with hemochromatosis including a liver transplantation program.

Support Groups
IDI's network of support-group coordinators is ever expanding. Coordinators are credentialed professionals such as registered nurses, physician's assistants, genetics counselors, MD's, teachers, or licensed nutritionists. Our concern is that the public receives answers to their questions from trained professionals, rather than individuals who are not medically qualified to address questions. Foremost is the health and well-being of individuals with disorders of iron. We encourage people to take charge of their health but to approach matters well informed and not to take action based on an emotionally charged event.

"Read, listen, think it through, then take action."

31
Role of Government Health Agencies

Reimbursement guidelines for physicians, provision of funding for research and development of new therapies are some of the ways our government health agencies influence health care. Every U.S. citizen is affected by what these agencies do, whether we have private insurance or not. Knowing about how our government health agencies function will help bring about a better understanding of how these agencies contribute to the health and well-being of every U.S. citizen.

Tax dollars are allocated by Congress to the different health agencies. Reimbursement guidelines are developed by the Health Care Finance Administration (HCFA) for Medicare. Physicians must follow these guidelines to get reimbursed for services including cost of laboratory tests. Research that is funded through the U.S. government is available in the form of grants, which scientists apply for periodically during the year. Grants are awarded on merit. The U.S. Department of Health and Human Services is by far the largest grant-producing agency in America, sending out over 60,000 grants per year.

U.S. Department of Health and Human Services
The guardian of U.S. health begins with the Secretary of Health and U.S. Surgeon General. "Early detection of iron overload disease (such as hemochromatosis) represents a major chronic disease prevention opportunity. Detection and treatment (phlebotomy) for iron overload early in the course of the illness can substantially

reduce the severity of the symptoms, organ damage and death from associated chronic disease, " says Assistant Secretary of Health and U.S. Surgeon General, David Satcher, M.D., Ph.D.

The United States Department of Health and Human Services is comprised of twelve operating divisions:
1. Office of the Surgeon General
2. Agency for Healthcare Research and Quality
3. Agency for Toxic Substances and Disease Registry
4. Administration on Aging
5. Administration for Children and Families
6. The Centers for Disease Control and Prevention
7. Food and Drug Administration
8. Health Care Financing Administration
9. Health Resources and Services Administration
10. Indian Health Service
11. he National Institutes of Health
12. Substance Abuse and Mental Health Services Administration

Each operating division contributes in some way to the health and well-being of a hemochromatosis patient. Emphasis in this section is on two key operating divisions that are directly funding research for HHC or developing educational materials and programs: the U.S. Centers for Disease Control and Prevention and the National Institutes of Health.

The U.S. Centers for Disease Control and Prevention
The CDC changed its name in 1970 from the Communicable Disease Center to the U.S. Centers for Disease Control and Prevention. CDC scientists were poised to accept new challenges. Among these were the deadly Ebola virus, sexually transmitted diseases including AIDS, hepatitis B and C, risks for breast, cervical, and ovarian cancers, and the prevention of chronic diseases, such as those associated with hemochromatosis.

CDC Mission: To promote health and quality of life by preventing and controlling disease, injury, and disability.

The CDC provides many of the administrative functions for the Agency for Toxic Substances and Disease Registry (ATSDR), a sister agency of CDC, and one of eight federal public health agencies within the Department of Health and Human Services.

The Director of CDC also serves as the administrator of ATSDR.
    Office of the Director: Dr. Jeffery Koplan
    Associate Director for Minority Health
    Associate Director for Science
    Freedom of Information Act Office
    Information Resources Management Office
    Management Analysis and Services Office
    National Vaccine Program Office
    Office of Communication, Division of Media Relations
    Office of Global Health
    Office of Health and Safety (OhASIS)
    Office of Women's Health
    Technology Transfer Office
    Washington, D.C., Office

- Epidemiology Program Office
- National Center for Chronic Disease Prevention and Health Promotion-Division of Nutrition and Physical Activity
- National Center for Environmental Health
- Office of Genetics and Disease Prevention
- National Center for Health Statistics
- National Center for HIV, STD, and TB Prevention
- National Center for Infectious Diseases
- National Center for Injury Prevention and Control
- National Immunization Program
- National Institute for Occupational Safety and Health
- Public Health Practice Program Office

Since 1996, the National Center for Chronic Disease Prevention and Health Promotion—Division of Nutrition and Physical Activity is where the majority of issues about hemochromatosis are addressed. The current division director, Dr. William Dietz, and the Hemochromatosis Team leader, Dr. Michele Reyes, lead a multidisciplinary team of experts in CDC's HHC program activities. These include:

- Better characterizing the prevalence of iron overload due to hereditary hemochromatosis and its associated morbidity and morality in the U.S.;
- Developing key teaching messages to educate health care providers and patients about early diagnosis and treatment for this condition;

- Promoting laboratory quality assurance for the identification of iron overload and the genetic mutations responsible for hemochromatosis;
- Assessing the usefulness of iron overload and genetic tests for diagnosis and screening.

Priorities
- Educating health care providers about early diagnosis and treatment of the disorder
- Promoting laboratory standardization and quality assurance for diagnostic tests to provide an evidence-based response to universal screening issues and recommendations for diagnostic test cut-points
- Improving the estimate of the prevalence of hemochromatosis and its associated morbidity and mortality in the U.S.
- Estimating the prevalence of iron overload within overload illnesses
- Describing the clinical course of the disorder
- Determining the risks and benefits of universal screening for early detection of hemochromatosis

Next Steps
CDC will launch its iron overload educational campaign for health care providers via the Internet, medical society meetings, scientific literature, and CDC publications. A downloadable (as well as hard copy) patient pamphlet on iron overload will also be available to health care providers for dissemination to their newly diagnosed patients. CDC will coordinate population-based studies to determine the prevalence and associated morbidity and mortality from hemochromatosis so that strategies for disease prevention can be developed. CDC will also begin to evaluate and quantify the potential benefits of early detection, characterize the consequences of undetected and untreated disease, and compare a variety of screening strategies for cost and benefit. In addition, CDC will further refine, standardize, and monitor laboratory tests and continue to enhance the education of health care providers on early diagnosis and treatment of hemochromatosis.

"CDC is very concerned about this known genetic disorder

because we now know hereditary hemochromatosis is common; we are armed with modern technology to recognize it early, and it is treatable. Our top priority for hemochromatosis at this time is education. We want to heighten the awareness of HH among health care providers, as well as the general population. We recommend that individuals experiencing unexplained symptoms (e.g., fatigue, joint pain, abdominal pain impotence, loss of menstruation, etc.) as well as certain medical problems (e.g., cirrhosis, liver cancer, diabetes, arthritis heart disease, etc.) speak with their health care provider about evaluation for hemochromatosis," says Michele Reyes, Ph.D. Hemochromatosis Team Leader, Chronic Disease and Nutrition Branch, Division of Nutrition and Physical Activity, US Centers for Disease Control and Prevention.

> "IT IS CLEAR THAT WE NEED TO HEIGHTEN HEALTH CARE PROVIDER AWARENESS (ABOUT IRON OVERLOAD DISEASE). WE NEED TO AT LEAST GET THEM THINKING ABOUT DOING TRANSFERRIN SATURATIONS IN PATIENTS WHO HAVE THESE KINDS OF EARLY NONSPECIFIC SYMPTOMS SO THAT PEOPLE ARE IDENTIFIED EARLY IN THE COURSE OF THE DISEASE RATHER THAN LATER WHEN THEY HAVE ALREADY DEVELOPED SYMPTOMS OR DISABILITY AND CERTAINLY WE NEED TO IDENTIFY THEM BEFORE THEY DEVELOP THIS LATE STAGE DISEASE."
>
> —*William Dietz, M.D., Director, Division of Nutrition and Physical Activity, NCCDPHP/CDC*

Office of Genetics and Disease Prevention

Muin J. Khoury, M.D., Ph.D., Director

The Office of Genetics and Disease Prevention was created by the Centers for Disease Control and Prevention in 1997 to help integrate advances in human genetics into public health research, policy and program development, and evaluation.

The Office of Genetics accomplishments include:

1. Representing the CDC at the Secretary of Health and Human Services Donna Shalala Advisory Committee on Genetic Testing (SACGT). This committee dovetails efforts with other agencies such as the Human Genome Research Institute and Alliance for Genetic Support Groups. Iron Disorders Institute Chairman and President Randy S. Alexander is

a participant on this committee.

SACGT will advise the government about all aspects of the development and use of genetic tests, including the complex medical, ethical, legal, and social issues raised by genetic testing. Among the general issues that the committee may take up include: the development of guidelines, including criteria regarding the risks and benefits of genetic testing, to assist institutional review boards in reviewing genetic testing protocols in both academic and commercial settings; the adequacy of regulatory oversight of genetic tests; provisions for assuring the quality of genetic testing laboratories; the need for mechanisms to track the introduction of genetic tests to enable accuracy and clinical effectiveness over time to be evaluated; and safeguarding the privacy and confidentiality of genetic information and preventing discrimination and stigmatization based on genetic information. Procedurally, recommendations made by the committee will be submitted to the Secretary through the Assistant Secretary for Health.

2. Promoting national leadership in genetics and public health by sponsoring public health working groups and the annual national conference on genetics and public health

3. Funding prevention research projects to assess how genetic information can be used to improve health and prevent disease

4. Funding a model system for collecting, analyzing, and disseminating data on genetic tests

5. Disseminating information on the impact of gene discoveries on disease prevention and public health

6. Providing training opportunities in genetics and public health

The National Institutes of Health
Begun as a one-room Laboratory of Hygiene in 1887, the National Institutes of Health today is one of the world's foremost medical research centers, and the Federal focal point for medical research in the U.S. Located in Bethesda, MD, and Triangle Park, North Carolina, the NIH is one of eight health agencies of the Public Health Services. It is comprised of 25 separate institutes and centers; those located in Bethesda are spread over 300 acres

contained within 75 buildings.

The various institutes are:

- Office of the Director
- National Institute on Aging (NIA)
- National Institute on Alcohol Abuse and Alcoholism (NIAAA)
- National Institute of Allergy and Infectious Diseases (NIAID
- National Institute of Arthritis and Musculoskeletal and Skin Diseases (NIAMS)
- National Cancer Institute (NCI)
- National Center for Complementary and Alternative Medicine (NCCAM)
- National Institute of Child Health and Human Development (NICHHD)
- National Institute on Deafness and Other Communication Disorders (NIDCD)
- National Institute of Dental and Craniofacial Research (NIDCR)
- The National Institute of Diabetes and Digestive and Kidney Diseases (NIDDK)
- National Institute on Drug Abuse (NIDA)
- National Institute of Environmental Health Sciences (NIEHS)
- National Eye Institute (NEI)
- National Institute of General Medical Sciences (NIGMS)
- National Heart, Lung, and Blood Institute (NHLBI)
- National Human Genome Research Institute (NHGRI)
- National Center for Information Technology
- National Institute of Mental Health (NIMH)
- National Institute of Neurological Disorders and Stroke (NINDS)
- National Institute of Nursing Research
- National Library of Medicine
- Warren Grant Magnuson Clinical Center
- Fogarty International Center (FIC)
- Center for Scientific Review (CSR)

While many institutes are funding directly or indirectly hemochromatosis and iron-related disease research, the following four are most prominent in their funding efforts for this disorder:

The National Institute of Diabetes and Digestive and Kidney Diseases

"Hereditary hemochromatosis is the most common genetic mutation known in the United States. The excessive iron accumulation in patients with the full-blown disease results in liver and heart failure, as well as diabetes and other ailments. Diagnosis has been a major problem, but the recent discovery of the gene, HFE, responsible for most cases of hereditary hemochromatosis, has revolutionized the opportunity both to understand and diagnose this genetic disorder. Clinical and basic science investigators are engaged in an intensive study of its cause and pathology. As a model genetic disease, hemochromatosis also will help us learn how to apply genetic knowledge to patient care and how to deal with societal implications of genetic diseases."—David G. Badman, Ph.D.

Hematology Program Director

Deputy Director for Basic Program Administration

DKUHD, NIDDK, NIH

The NIDDK conducts and supports much of the clinical research on the diseases of internal medicine and related subspecialty fields as well as many basic science disciplines. The institute's Division of Intramural Research encompasses the broad spectrum of metabolic diseases such as diabetes, inborn errors of metabolism, endocrine disorders, mineral metabolism, digestive diseases, nutrition, urology and renal disease, and hematology. Basic research studies include biochemistry, nutrition, pathology, histochemistry, chemistry, physical, chemical, and molecular biology, pharmacology, and toxicology.

NIDDK extramural research is organized into divisions of program areas: Division of Diabetes, Endocrinology, and Metabolic Diseases.

DEM provides research funding and support for basic and clinical research in the areas of type 1 and type 2 diabetes and other metabolic disorders, including cystic fibrosis; endocrinology and endocrine disorders; obesity, neuroendocrinology, and energy balance; and development, metabolism, and basic biology of liver, fat, and endocrine tissues. DEM also provides funding for the training and career development of individuals committed to academic and clinical research careers in these areas.

Division of Digestive Diseases and Nutrition

DDN has responsibility for managing programs in basic and clinical research, as well as training and career development, related to liver and biliary diseases; pancreatic diseases; gastrointestinal disease, including neuroendocrinology, motility, immunology, absorption, and transport in the gastrointestinal tract; nutrient metabolism; obesity; and eating disorders.

Division of Kidney, Urologic, and Hematologic Diseases

KUH provides research funding and support for basic and clinical research in the areas of kidney diseases including end-stage renal disease, kidney disease of diabetes, IgA nephropathy, hemolytic uremic syndrome, polycystic kidney disease, hypertensive nephrosclerosis, acute renal failure and fluid and electrolyte disorders; urinary tract diseases including benign prostatic hyperplasia, urinary tract infections, kidney stones, impotence, urinary incontinence, and interstitial cystitis; and disorders of the blood and blood-forming organs.

Current hemochromatosis research underway funded by the NIDDK:

Penn State College of Medicine: to determine how the hemochromatosis protein normally controls iron absorption within the intestine. Humans have an automatic iron regulation mechanism. In people with normal iron metabolism, this system allows us to take in more iron when needs are great such as growth spurts, blood loss, and trauma. This same system can reduce the amount of dietary iron absorbed when chronic illness is present. For those with hemochromatosis, an inborn error of metabolism, this regulatory process may contribute to excessive absorption of iron. This study will contribute to a better understanding of iron regulation in the gut.

Principal investigators are: Dr. James R. Connor of the Department of Neuroscience and Anatomy and colleagues Dr. Jing Hu and Dr. Harriet C. Isom of the Departments of Microbiology and Immunology and Pathology, Dr. Edward E. Cable, Research Associate, Dr. Michael J. Chorney of the Departments of Microbiology and Immunology and Pediatrics, Dr. John Beard of the Nutrition Department, and Dr. Mel Billingsley of the Department of Pharmacology and Director of Hershey's Macromolecular Core Facility.

Kaiser Permanente/Scripps Research Institute: to determine the gene frequency of the three HFE mutations (C282Y, H63D, S65C) and to relate genotypes to various clinical and laboratory values in 10,198 adults.

Principal investigators: Drs. Ernest Beutler, Vincent Felitti, Terri Gelbart, and Ngoc Ho

The research program was begun in 1997 as a joint project with Dr. E. Beutler, Scripps Research Center and Dr. V. Felitti, Kaiser Permanente and funded with two grants from the NIDDK, and supplemented with a grant from the Centers for Disease Control and Prevention, and Stein Endowment Fund. Results of their observational study are published in 5 September 2000 *Annals of Internal Medicine* Vol. 133: Number 5 entitled: The Effect of HFE Geneotypes on Measurements of Iron Overload in Patients Attending a Health Appraisal Clinic, Reprints are available through Barbara Hudson Reprints Coordinator 215-351-2657 or by email to bhudson@mail.acponline.org

The National Heart, Lung, and Blood Institute
The National Heart, Lung, and Blood Institute (NHLBI) provides leadership for a national program in diseases of the heart, blood vessels, lung, and blood; blood resources; and sleep disorders.

The Institute plans, conducts, fosters, and supports an integrated and coordinated program of basic research, clinical investigations and trials, observational studies, and demonstration and education projects. Research is related to the causes, prevention, diagnosis, and treatment of heart, blood vessel, lung, and blood diseases; and sleep disorders. The NHLBI plans and directs research in development and evaluation of interventions and devices related to prevention, treatment, and rehabilitation of patients suffering from such diseases and disorders. It also supports research on clinical use of blood and all aspects of the management of blood resources. Research is conducted in the institute's own laboratories and by scientific institutions and individuals supported by research grants and contracts. For health professionals and the public, the NHLBI conducts educational activities, including development and dissemination of materials in the above areas, with an emphasis on prevention.

The NHLBI supports research training and career development of new and established researchers in fundamental sciences and clinical disciplines to enable them to conduct basic and clinical research related to heart, blood vessel, lung, and blood diseases; sleep disorders; and blood resources through individual and institutional research training awards and career development awards.

The institute coordinates relevant activities in the above areas, including the related causes of stroke, with other research institutes and federal health programs. Relationships are maintained with institutions and professional associations, and with international, national, state, and local officials as well as voluntary agencies and organizations working in the above areas.

> "HEMOCHROMATOSIS IS ONE OF THE MOST COMMON INHERITED DISORDERS AND ONE THAT IS EASILY TREATABLE IF DIAGNOSED EARLY. UNFORTUNATELY, EARLY DIAGNOSIS IS DIFFICULT AND TOO OFTEN THE DISEASE IS NOT DETECTED UNTIL SEVERE COMPLICATIONS HAVE OCCURRED. EARLY DIAGNOSIS HAS THE POTENTIAL TO ONE DAY ELIMINATE THE ORGAN DAMAGE AND OTHER LIFE-THREATENING COMPLICATIONS NOW SUFFERED BY THOSE WITH HEMOCHROMATOSIS."
>
> —*Dr. Claude Lenfant,*
> *Director of the NHLBI*

National Human Genome Research Institute (NHGRI)

The NHGRI was originally established in 1989 as The National Center for Human Genome Research (NCHGR). Its mission is to head the Human Genome Project for the National Institutes of Health (NIH). The NHGRI is one of twenty-five institutes, centers, or divisions that make up the NIH, the federal government's primary agency for the support of biomedical research. The collective research components of the NIH make up the largest biomedical research facility in the world. The NIH is part of the U.S. Department of Health and Human Services and funded by tax dollars.

The NHGRI set as its goal to complete the sequence of the entire human genome by 2003. To accomplish this monumental task, they formed a consortium of sixteen institutions in France, Germany, Japan, China, Great Britain, and the United States. The five largest centers are located at Baylor College of Medicine, Houston, Texas; Joint Genome Institute, Walnut Creek, California; the Sanger Centre near Cambridge, England; Washington University School of Medicine, St. Louis; and Whitehead Institute, Cambridge, Massachusetts. Originally estimated to cost $3 billion and take fifteen years to complete (1990–2005), by June 2000 a working draft was available at the cost of $300 million. Half, or $150 million, was funded by the NIH.

> "THE HUMAN GENOME PROJECT EFFORT IS TO READ THE ENTIRE SEQUENCE OF ALL THE HUMAN DNA BY THE YEAR 2005. IT'S AN INTERNATIONAL EFFORT, BUT THE UNITED STATES HAS THE SCIENTIFIC LEAD ON THIS, AND AS THE DIRECTOR OF THE NATIONAL HUMAN GENOME RESEARCH INSTITUTE, WHICH IS PART OF THE NATIONAL INSTITUTES OF HEALTH. IT IS MY JOB, TO OVERSEE THIS EFFORT."
>
> —*Francis Collins, M.D., Ph.D., Director, Human Genome Research Institute*

NHLBI/NHGRI are jointly funding a multicenter, multiethnic, primary care–based sample of 100,000 adults in a five-year study to determine the epidemiology of HFE prevalence, genetic and environmental determinants, and potential clinical, personal, and societal impact of iron overload and hereditary hemochromatosis.

Contributing centers: Field Centers: Ronald Acton, M.D., University of Alabama; Paul Adams, M.D., London Health Sciences Centre, London, Ontario, Canada; Victor Gordeuk, M.D., Howard University; Christine McLaren, Ph.D., University of California, Irvine; and Emily Harris, Ph.D., Kaiser Permanente Center for Health Research, Portland. Central Lab: John Eckfeldt, M.D., Ph.D., University of Minnesota. Data Coordinating Center: David Reboussin, Ph.D., Wake Forrest.

Individuals who are genetically tested can be victims of discrimination. Data from this study will serve as the framework for the Advisory Committee on Genetic Testing (SACGT) policy guidelines that will be submitted to the Secretary of Health and

Human Services, Donna Shalala, for approval and potential legislation to protect the health and well-being of U.S. citizens against discrimination as a result of genetic testing outcome.

This research project was born out of a workshop, cosponsored by the Centers for Disease Control and Prevention (CDC) and NHGRI, held March 3, 1997, to examine the clinical, ethical, legal, and social implications of discovery of the gene for hereditary hemochromatosis and the possibility of widespread population-based testing for the disease.

An article detailing the conclusions resulting from this workshop was published in the July 8, 1998 issue of *JAMA* (Wylie Burke et al., "Hereditary Hemochromatosis: Gene Discovery and Its Implications for Population-Based Screening" (pp. 172-78).

National Institute of Neurological Disorders and Stroke (NINDS)
Supports the study of stroke, sleep disorders, epilepsy, Alzheimer's, Parkinson's, multiple sclerosis, restless legs syndrome, ADD/ADHD, and depression, conditions known to be related to iron imbalances.

NINDS is providing grants for three different research projects with principal investigators Drs. James Connor, Department of Neuroscience and Anatomy, and John Beard, Department of Nutrition, Penn State University. There is a known link with iron to such neurological-related problems as Alzheimer's, early onset Parkinson's, ADD/ADHD, depression, epilepsy, hypothyroidism, and hypogonadism. These three critically important research projects will be helpful in understanding the mechanisms by which iron influences these illnesses. The three research programs are to study the dynamics of iron transport into the brain to determine the role of iron in the outcome of infants who are hypoxic/ischemic at birth and to determine if the brain regulates iron uptake, and if so, how?

All government health agencies are funded by U.S. tax dollars specifically allocated to these various agencies. Nearly 20 percent of the total U.S. budget is distributed among these entities.

In conclusion
Anyone who wishes to have particular research funded needs to know how our government health agencies are funded. Congress

allocates funds to the NIH and CDC based on perceived need. IDI has endeavored to raise awareness about hemochromatosis among our legislators so that the CDC and NIH can continue to receive funding that allows them to do research and studies related to hemochromatosis. Your congressman or senator is the person to contact about these matters. Among those already aware include:

"Hemochromatosis is a disease that need not be fatal. Former Senator Connie Mack and I have worked for a long time to get Congress to recognize that this disease can be treated as a preventive health care issue. Through the appropriations process, we consistently urged the Centers for Disease Control to use congressional funding to expand its clinical screening efforts and educate physicians about hemochromatosis so that individuals can be diagnosed earlier and can begin combating this disease." —Ernest Fritz Hollings, United States Senate

"Early detection of Hemochromatosis offers a good opportunity to prevent chronic disease and early death . . ." —Connie Mack, United States Senate

"Hemochromatosis is a little known and sometimes overlooked disorder. I am pleased there is increasing public awareness about it. I believe a better understanding of both the symptoms and the prevalence of the disorder will help ensure that those with hemochromatosis will get an early diagnosis and the necessary medical treatment." —Jay Rockefeller, United States Senate

"Hereditary hemochromatosis is among the most common genetic disorders, which results in excess iron accumulation, tissue damage, and systematic organ failure. The Committee recognizes hereditary hemochromatosis as one of the most common genetic disorders. The committee notes CDC's efforts and encourages their continued progress in this area." —Fiscal Year 2000 House /Senate /Conference Appropriations Language

Commonly Asked Questions and Answers

Q: What is ng/mL?
A: nanograms/milliliter

Q: What is ug/L?
A: microgram/liter

Q: What is transferrin? And explain transferrin iron saturation percentage.
A: Transferrin is a protein that binds with iron and transports it to places within the body, such as bone marrow, liver and to ferritin. Transferrin is usually 25–35 percent saturated with iron, meaning it has about 65–70 percent capacity left to bind surplus iron. When transferrin is 100 percent saturated, a person is overloaded with iron. A corresponding elevated serum ferritin will accompany an elevated TS percent when tissue iron is high.

Q: What is UIBC?
A: Unsaturated iron-binding capacity; it is another way to determine iron overload.

Q: I have one copy of C282Y and one copy of H63D. My ferritin is 300.5 ug/L; I have normal liver enzymes, and do not have hepatomegaly. Would I be a candidate for liver biopsy?
A: Most scientists include the compound heterozygote (C282Y/H63D) in the same risk category as the C282Y homozygote and therefore, the same guidelines apply: "Patients

homozygous for the C282Y mutation for HFE, with ferritin levels less than 1000 ng/mL, and normal liver enzymes, and do not have hepatomegaly, are unlikely to have cirrhosis/fibrosis. Therefore these patients are not candidates for liver biopsy."—*idInsight*, 1st Quarter 1999

Q: I don't want to have a liver biopsy and I don't want to get the gene test but I have real high iron, is there another way to get my diagnosis?

A: Your physician can begin therapeutic phlebotomy; hemoglobins of individuals with iron overload will return to normal following the initial phases of de-ironing. Some refer to this means of diagnosis as quantitative phlebotomy.

Q: Hereditary hemochromatosis is HHC, correct?

A: Yes, depending upon where you live, you may see any one of the following acronyms for hemochromatosis: HHC refers to hereditary human hemochromatosis. HH is hereditary hemochromatosis, HC hemochromatosis, and GH genetic hemochromatosis.

Q: Sometimes I believe that hemochromatosis is used whenever iron overload is present and other times I think that hemochromatosis cannot be present unless it is hereditary. What is the correct definition for hemochromatosis?

A: Hereditary hemochromatosis is HFE-related; 90 percent of people with hemochromatosis have known HFE gene mutations. There are other kinds of iron overload disease where the HFE gene is not involved.

Q: With DNA testing, it can be determined if you have a single gene mutation (heterozygote), or double mutation (homozygote), or have a combination of gene mutations (compound heterozygote). Can a single gene mutation (heterozygote) be either C282Y or H63D?

A: Yes.

Q: Can a double mutation (homozygote) be either two copies of C282Y or two copies of H63D?

A: Yes—or any subsequently identified mutation.

Q: How many mutations of HFE are there?
A: No one knows. Currently there are several identified and known to result in iron overload: on chromosome 6 these include: C282S, H63D, S65C.

Q: Do any other chromosomes have mutations that can result in iron overload?
A: Yes, Dr. Clara Camaschella et al., have identified a mutation on chromosome 1: Y250X.

Q: A combination of gene mutations (compound heterozygote) must be one copy of C282Y and one copy of H63D?
A: Yes, one copy of two different mutations. There are now other mutations; S65C is one of them.

Q: Can any of these five situations be any worse than any of the others? If so, what is the order from the least desirable to the not so bad and how much difference is there between them?
A: This depends on penetrance or how a gene manifests itself in a person. Some C282Y homozygotes never get sick, others get very ill. Scientists don't know why.

Q: I have heard that genetic testing is done by PCR for the HFE mutation; what is PCR?
A: Polymerase chain reaction (used in making copies of genes for purpose of genetic testing).

Q: What is the difference between HFE gene and HLA-H gene?
A: HFE is the gene for hereditary hemochromatosis. HLA-H is tissue typing mostly used for transplantation purposes. Individuals with HHC have certain HLA-H characteristics specific enough to highly suspect hemochromatosis. HLA typing was used prior to discovery of HFE.

Q: Hereditary hemochromatosis affects one in 400 individuals of Northern European descent. The C282Y gene occurs in 1 in 8

Caucasians. So, out of 400 individuals, one has hemochromatosis but 50 have C282Y, correct? H63D gene occurs how often in 400 individuals?

A: Originally, the C282Y mutation is what the prevalence was based on. This was due in part to the belief that other mutations were not so significant as C282Y. Studies are under way to determine the importance of H63D, S65C, and other mutations being discovered such as C282S and X250Y. Worldwide HFE prevalence average is 1-250-300. In Ireland it is 1:80 and the southeastern region of the USA, HFE prevalence is 1:125.

Q: Must you have two defective genes in order to have hereditary hemochromatosis?

A: Yes, by the current definition, but you can have iron overload without HFE mutations.

Q: If one parent has one defective gene and the other parent is normal, will any of the children inherit one or more defective genes?

A: All children have a 50 percent chance of being a carrier. None has a chance of being homozygous because the mutations come in this way: one from father, one from mother.

Q: I have two defective genes, C282Y and H63D, but my wife is normal. Will any of our children inherit one or more defective genes?

A: Your children will be obligate heterozygotes or carriers but they may receive different mutations; that is, some will be C282Y carriers and some will be H63D carriers.

Q: My blood work was NOT done while I was fasting. Will this make a great deal of difference in the results?

A: Yes, a test done not fasting can cause a false positive on transferrin iron saturation percentage. Serum iron can be affected by several factors such as foods you have eaten. Serum iron is best measured following a fast.

Q: I have had a problem sleeping all my life. Is this associated with HHC?

A: Sleep-related problems such as waking in the middle of the night, sleep apnea, and insomnia are symptoms that might be associated with iron imbalances but not necessarily HHC. Iron imbalances such as iron deficiency anemia can cause restless legs syndrome, which can disrupt sleep.

Q: Could migraine headaches be associated with HHC?

A: Perhaps, some migraine are caused by hormonal imbalances. Individuals with HHC often have hormone imbalance symptoms.

Q: Can the use of magnets at any area of your body be harmful to patients with hemochromatosis?

A. Iron in your body is not magnetic. Magnets should not pose any greater threat to a person with HHC than any other person.

Q: Can young women age 25–30, experience arthritic conditions due to HHC prior to their showing any elevated iron retention?

A: Yes, early joint pain can be one of the first signs of hemochromatosis, possibly due to pituitary damage and hormone imbalances.

Q: Can this condition (HHC/iron overload) be misdiagnosed as other conditions such as psoriatic arthritis and influence the treatment?

A. Yes, determining the underlying cause of arthritic pain can be complicated. Arthritic pain for those with HHC is due to a pseudo-gout type condition where these individuals will test sero-negative for rheumatoid arthritis.

Q: What is the correct criteria for therapeutic phlebotomy? My doctor wants it done for Hgb 13. I have a ferritin level below normal, but Hgb is between 14 and 15.

A: Phlebotomy may be done when hematocrit is 34 percent or higher. There is no known benefit to ferritin levels less than 10 ng/mL.

Q: Has there been any such association made between iron and seizures/epilepsy?

A: Yes, excellent studies about brain iron and epilepsy are under way. Individuals with HHC have reported seizure episodes among symptoms they have experienced.

Q: Can iron load in animals?

A: Yes, this is called animalis siderosis. According to pathologist Dr. Donald Paglia, birds of paradise, crows, hornbills, mynahs, ostriches, quetzels, sparrow, starlings, tanager, toucans, lemurs, seals, and black rhinos are capable of getting iron overload. Read more about this in *idInsight,* spring issue 2001.

Q: Has there been any connection made between iron overload and neuropathy?

A: Yes, in diabetes and myalgias such as fibromyalgia.

Q: Any connection between tinnitus and/or impaired hearing and iron overload?

A: An excellent paper by Drs. Conlon and Smith addresses the issue of aminoglycoside antibiotics plus iron and hearing loss. There is evidence that this combination contributes to hearing loss. Read more about this in *idInsight,* spring issue 2001.

Q: After I was diagnosed with hemochromatosis it was determined that I also have sideroblastic anemia. I would welcome any counsel as to personal understanding and responsible handling of these two disorders.

A: Human trials are under way to test a new and promising therapeutic procedure that can remove iron outside the body using a chelating agent such as Desferal. This therapy is ideal for someone with concurrent iron overload and anemia. Write to the Iron Disorders Institute for updates on this therapy.

Q: I do not have the genetic component, so can I get iron overload from food or supplements?

A: If you have normal iron metabolism your body will regulate how much iron you absorb. You might just get an upset stomach. However, you could have one of the undiscovered gene mutations that result in abnormal iron absorption and therefore be at risk. Also, you can inhale iron in tobacco smoke and misusers of alcohol will absorb greater amounts of iron. Obtained this way it matters not that you have normal or abnormal metabolism. Inhaled iron bypasses that regulatory process. It is best not to supplement unless hemoglobin values and underlying causes of anemia indicate supplementation is appropriate.

Q: Is it possible to have hemochromatosis and have normal iron levels (TIBC, UIBC, iron sat, ferritin and iron serum)? I have recently had a CT of the chest and it showed my liver to be markedly hyperdense, indicative of hemochromatosis, yet, my iron studies were normal.

A: Yes, it is possible for you to have tests in the "normal range" and yet have HHC.

Q: I have had some of the symptoms of hemochromatosis, e.g., fatigue, weight loss, chest pain, and right upper quadrant pain. I am scheduled to have an MRI of the liver and I have ordered a DNA test. What else should I have?

A: Serum iron, TIBC, and serum ferritin, preferably measured fasting.

Glossary of Terms

acidosis: a condition resulting from accumulation of too much acid in the body due to excess carbon dioxide; acidic individuals may sigh frequently, have insomnia, or migraines. Neutral pH is 7.0, above 7.0 is alkaline, below 7.0 is acidic. Ideal body pH is around 7.4.

ACTH (adrenocorticotropic hormone): hormone secreted by the anterior pituitary gland, which stimulates adrenal glands to secrete the hormones such as cortisone, the body's natural pain-reliever. ACTH is secreted during moments of stress, trauma, major surgery, and fever.

acute: occurring suddenly and severely but of short duration; can define pain as sharp.

Addison's disease or syndrome (adrenal insufficiency): inactive or underactive adrenal glands. Symptoms might include weakness, fatigue, weight loss, low blood pressure, behavior changes, abdominal pain, diarrhea, appetite loss, cold intolerance, brown-colored skin, disturbance in glucose levels, electrolyte and mineral imbalances.

adhesions: bands of fibrous tissue that cause organs to abnormally bind together, most commonly found in the abdomen frequently following surgery. Can cause abdominal pain.

adrenal gland: a pair of triangle shaped ductless hormone glands that rest above the kidneys; part of the endocrine system. Adrenal cortex is the outer layer of the adrenal gland where various hormones including cortisone, estrogen, testosterone, cortisol, androgen, aldosterone and progesterone are secreted. Adrenal medulla is the middle part of the adrenal gland that secretes epinephrine (same as adrenaline) and the neurotransmitter norepinephrine.

Adrenal insufficiency: *see* Addison's disease.

advanced directive: written instructions as in a living will required by federal law whereby all hospitalized patients have a form on file indicating their desires.

AIDS (Acquired Immune Deficiency Syndrome): usually fatal condition whereby the immune system loses the ability to fight infection or suppress multiplication of abnormal cells, such as cancer cells. Virus is derived from contaminated blood, sexual contact with infected person, syringe used by infected person, or from an infected mother who passes the virus to a fetus.

aldosterone: a powerful hormone excreted by the adrenal gland; indirectly regulates blood levels of potassium and chloride, among others, a well as Ph, blood volume, and blood pressure.

alkalosis: abnormal condition in which body fluids are more alkaline than normal. Symptoms may include abdominal pain, diarrhea, loss of appetite, and brown skin. Caused by conditions that decrease the level of carbon dioxide in the blood, such as prolonged vomiting, excess intake of bicarbonate, breathing too rapidly, or congestive heart failure. *See* congestive heart failure.

ALP (alkaline phosphatase): Liver enzyme that can concentrate in liver and bone. Increased levels may show as cirrhosis, primary or metastatic liver tumor, or biliary obstruction.

alpha-fetoprotein (AFP): dominant oncofetal protein produced by fetal liver and yolk sac during first trimester. Increased maternal serum levels may indicate neural tube or abdominal wall defects in the fetus. Increased nonmaternal AFP may indicate hepatoma or other cancers or liver cell necrocis.

ALT (alanine aminotransferase): Liver enzyme (also see SGPT) that can concentrate in muscles, liver, and brain. Increased levels indicate cell death or disease in these tissues.

alveolus (alveoli, pl. of alveolus): tiny air sacs in the lungs where the exchange of carbon dioxide and oxygen occurs.

Alzheimer's disease: Named for Alois Alzheimer, neurologist, 1864–1915; a chronic, progressive disorder that accounts for more than 50 percent of all cases of dementia.

amenorrhea: cessation of menstruation for at least three months in a woman who has previously menstruated. Causes include pregnancy, breastfeeding, eating disorders, endocrine disorders, psychological disorders, menopause (usually thirty-five years of age or older), surgical removal of uterus or ovaries, or very strenuous athletic activities.

amino acids: organic compounds mostly made of proteins. The body contains at least twenty amino acids; ten are essential. The body doesn't make or form these, so they must be acquired through diet.

amylase: a type of enzyme that splits starches; classed as either alpha (found in animals) or beta (found in plants).

amyloidosis: disorder in which starchlike glycoproteins (amyloids) accumulate in tissues, impairing function.

ANA (antinuclear antibody): used to diagnose systemic lupus erythematosus, a chronic inflammatory disease.

androstenedione: hormone; precursor of testosterone and estrogen. Increased levels may indicate adrenal tumor or congenital adrenal hyperplasia.

anemia: condition in which the iron needs exceed the iron content of the blood. See anemia of chronic disease, aplastic, Cooley's, Falconi's, hemolytic, iron deficiency anemia, pernicious, peroxidine (B6 deficiency) dependent, sickle cell, sideroblastic, thalassemia.

anemia, aplastic: serious disease caused by a failure of the bone marrow to produce blood cells. Symptoms may include paleness, weakness, bleeding from the nose, mouth, rectum, as well as internally, frequent infection, unexplained bruising, May be caused by neoplasm (tumor) or destruction of the bone marrow by exposure to certain chemicals, anticancer drugs, immunosuppressive drugs, or antibiotics. Cause is sometimes unknown. Curable if cause can be identified and treated successfully.

anemia, Cooley's (also known as thalassemia): inherited disorder where a recessive trait is responsible for interference with hemoglobin synthesis.

anemia of chronic disease: mild anemia that accompanies inflammation due to chronic disease.

anemia, Falconi's (also known as Falconi's syndrome): rare type anemia, usually congenital disorder characterized by aplastic anemia, bone abnormalities, olive-brown skin pigmentation, abnormally small head, small gonads, and kidney-function abnormalities. When found in children the child usually develops severe aplastic anemia by age eight to nine years. Treatment usually consists of bone marrow transplantation. Adults can get a form of the syndrome as a result of heavy-metal poisoning. It also may occur after a kidney transplant.

anemia, hemolytic: inherited disorder where premature destruction of mature red blood cells occurs.

anemia, iron deficiency: anemia caused by blood loss, dietary insufficiencies, or rapid growth where iron demands exceed intake and stores.

anemia, pernicious: anemia caused by inadequate absorption of vitamin B_{12} due to the absence of intrinsic factor, a substance secreted by the mucous membranes of the stomach.

anemia, pyridoxine-responsive: decreased red blood cells in circulation, which increase to normal with pyridoxine (B_6) treatment.

anemia, sickle cell: severe, incurable anemia that occurs in people who have an abnormal form of hemoglobin in their blood cells. It is an inherited disease and derives its name from the sickle-shaped cells that are present with this disorder.

anemia, sideroblastic: type of anemia in which the bone marrow deposits iron prematurely into red blood cells. These cells do not transport oxygen to the body as efficiently as normal cells.

anemia, thalassemia major: see anemia, Cooley's.

angina: chest pain or pressure usually beneath the sternum (breastbone). Caused by inadequate blood supply to the heart. Often brought on by exercise, emotional upset, or heavy meals in someone who has heart disease.

angiogardiography: cardiac catheterization used to visualize the heart chambers, arteries, and veins.

angiography (also called arteriography): an x-ray technique. Radiopaque contrast material is injected into the desired artery during x-ray filming. Blood-flow abnormalities and tumors can be easily seen using this procedure.

angiomas: benign tumors, usually congenital, made up of mostly blood vessels or lymph vessels.

angioplasty: the use of surgery to make a damaged blood vessel function properly again; may involve widening or reconstructing the blood vessel.

angiotension-converting enzyme (ACE) inhibitor: a drug used to decrease pressure inside blood vessels.

antibody: a protein made by white blood cells that reacts with a specific foreign protein as part of the immune response.

antidiuretic: substance that controls the amount of water reabsorbed by the kidney.

apheresis: a therapeutic procedure. The blood is filtered, during which time the red blood cells or other blood components are removed. Can be used to treat conditions such as iron overload or sickle-cell anemia.

arrhythmia: an irregular heartbeat, may be rapid or seeming to skip beats.

arthritis: inflammatory condition of the joints, characterized by pain, stiffness, and swelling; see rheumatoid and sero-negative rheumatoid arthritis.

arthrography/arthrogram: x-ray of a joint with contrast dye.

arthropathy: any joint disease.

arthroscopy: a procedure that allows direct examination of the interior of a joint using a specially designed instrument.

ascites: accumulation of fluid in the abdomen; may be a complication of cirrhosis, congestive heart failure, kidney malfunction, cancer, peritonitis, or various fungal and parasitic diseases.

aspiration: withdrawal by suction of fluids, air or foreign bodies.

AST (aspartate aminotransferase): a liver enzyme concentrated in the muscles, liver, and brain. Increased levels may indicate liver diseases such as hepatitis, cirrhosis, tumors, etc.

atherosclerosis: common disorder of the arteries characterized by thickening, loss of elasticity, and calcification of artery walls. Results in decreased blood supply to the brain and lower extremities. Typical signs include pain on walking, poor circulation in feet and legs, headache, dizziness, and memory defects.

autoimmune disease: a disorder in which the body's immune system attacks itself.

autoimmune thyroiditis: chronic inflammation that can lead to Grave's disease (hyperthyroidism) or hypothyroidism if the thyroid gland diminishes in size. See Grave's disease; hypothyroidism.

bacteria: plural of bacterium.

bacterium: a tiny, single-celled microorganism, commonly known as a germ; some bacteria, called pathogens, cause disease.

benign: harmless noncancerous tumor or growth that does not interfere with normal function.

beta-blocker: a drug used to treat hypertension (high blood pressure), heart arrhythmia, circulation, and sometimes angina or migraines. Drug slows the heart rate and reduces pressure inside blood vessels. Beta-blockers can also regulate heart rhythm.

bile duct: connects and conducts bile from the liver to the hepatic duct; joins the duct from the gall bladder to form the common bile duct.

biliary disease cirrhosis: a form of liver cirrhosis marked by enlargement of the liver and jaundice.

bilirubin: red blood cell waste product in bile, orange-yellowish in color; blood carries it to the liver. It contributes to the yellow color of urine. Jaundice occurs with abnormal accumulation of bilirubin in the blood and skin. Increased bilirubin level may also be involved in extensive liver damage.

biopsy: removal of a small amount of tissue or fluid, usually by needle, for laboratory examination; aids in diagnosis.

bleeding, gastrointestinal: condition of internal blood loss occurring somewhere in the digestive system—esophagus, stomach, small and large intestines.

blood: liquid pumped by the heart through arteries, veins, and capillaries. It consists of a pale yellow fluid called plasma, red blood cells (erythrocytes), white blood cells (leukocytes), platelets (thrombocyte—essential blood clotting element), and suspended chemicals, hormones, proteins, fats, and carbohydrates. Men have about 70 ml/kg of body weight and women about 65 ml/kg. *See* plasma. Blood's major function is to transport oxygen and nutrients to cells and remove from cells carbon dioxide and other waste products for detoxification and elimination.

blood pressure: measure of tension caused by blood pressing against the walls of the arteries as it flows through the body.

blood sugar: measure of glucose in the blood.

blood test: a lab procedure. Blood is drawn and tests made to determine the chemical or serum components or characteristics of the whole blood or some part of it.

bone marrow: specialized soft tissue that fills the core of bones. Most of the body's red and white blood cells are produced in bone marrow.

bone marrow aspiration: removal of a portion of the soft organic material filling the cavities of the bone. Used to evaluate and diagnose many blood diseases such as anemia, leukemia, iron storage deficiency, bone marrow deficiencies, or identification of tumors.

brain infarctions: localized area of brain tissue death resulting from lack of oxygen to that area because of an interruption in blood supply. Severity of symptoms following brain infarction depends on the location of the infarct and the extent of damage. *See* infarction.

breast cancer: a malignancy of the breast.

BUN (Blood Urea Nitrogen): a blood test. The BUN levels relates to the level of both liver and kidney function.

calcification: when the mineral calcium contained in the blood is deposited into tissues from injury, infection or aging. Often it is part of healing and not a sign of active disease but can lead to impaired organ function such as in kidneys and arteries.

calcium: mineral contained in the blood that helps regulate the heartbeat, transmit nerve impulses, contract muscles, and form bones and teeth.

calcium channel blocker (CCB): a drug used to relax the blood vessel and heart muscle, causing pressure inside blood vessels to drop. CCB drugs can be used to regulate heart rhythm.

cancer: abnormal and malignant growth of cells that invade nearby tissues, often spreading (metastasizing); also called carcinoma.

candida: a common bowel yeast, *Candida albicans*.

cardiac arrest: a sudden stop of heart function. See "sudden death"

cardiac catheterization: a procedure in which a thin hollow tube is inserted into a blood vessel. The tube is then advanced through the vessel into the heart, enabling a physician to study the heart and its pumping activity.

cardiac enzymes: an enzyme found in the heart muscle; when elevated indicates injury to the heart or skeletal muscle or possibly the brain.

cardiomyopathy disease: weakens the heart muscle so that the heart cannot efficiently pump blood. May be curable if the underlying cause is curable such as quitting smoking or drinking.

celiac disease: congenital (present at birth) disorder caused by an intolerance for gluten, a protein present in most grains. Gluten triggers an allergic reaction in the small intestine, which prevents the intestine from absorbing nutrients. Symptoms include poor appetite, abdominal bloating, fatigue, and pale, bad-smelling stool that floats on water. Treatment includes a high-protein, high-calorie, gluten-free diet and vitamin-mineral supplements. Recovery is usually complete with treatment.

cerebrospinal fluid: a clear, normally colorless and blood-free fluid acting as a cushion to protect the brain and spinal cord from injury.

ceruloplasmin (Cp): a blood glycoprotien; most of the copper in the blood is attached to it. An increased Cp level may indicate biliary cirrhosis or infection, while decreased Cp level may indicate Wilson's disease.

chemotherapy: treatment of cancer with medication intended to kill cancer cells without harming healthy tissue. Used to treat cancers that cannot be completely cured or treated with surgery or radiation.

cholesterol: complex chemical present in all animal fats. Cholesterol attaches to lipoproteins in the blood; low-density lipoproteins (LDL) carry cholesterol that builds up plaque; high-density lipoproteins (HDL) carry cholesterol to the liver where the body can get rid of it.

chromosome: structures inside the nucleus of living cells that contain hereditary information. Defects in chromosomes cause many birth defects and inherited diseases.

chronic: long-term; continuing. Chronic illnesses are usually not curable, but they can often be prevented from worsening by controlling symptoms.

cirrhosis: a chronic disease of the liver causing loss of function of liver cells and decreased blood flow through the liver.

colitis: inflammatory condition of the large intestine. It can occur in episodes, such as irritable bowel syndrome, or it can be one of the more serious, chronic, progressive, inflammatory bowel diseases, such as ulcerative colitis. *See* ulcerative colitis. Irritable bowel syndrome is characterized by bouts of colicky abdominal pain, bloating, diarrhea or constipation, and fatigue, often due to emotional stress. Treatment includes stress reduction, diet changes, and sometimes medication.

colonoscopy: investigation of the inside of the colon using a long, flexible fiberoptic tube.

complete blood count (CBC): The number of red corpuscles and white blood cells in a given measure of blood. A CBC will determine hemoglobin and hematocrit counts.

computed tomography (CT): a more precise x-ray measurement using computer analysis of the plane of the body selected. *See* tomography.

congenital: present at, and existing from, the time of birth.

congestion: abnormal fluid accumulation in the body, especially the lungs.

congestive heart failure: abnormal condition where the heart loses its full pumping capacity; fluid accumulates in the lungs causing shortness of breath. Usually accompanied by fatigue, and edema (abnormal accumulation of fluid in body tissues) in the extremities.

connective-tissue disease (collagen disease): any one of many abnormal conditions characterized by inflammatory changes in small blood vessels and connective tissue. Some collagen diseases include systemic lupus erythematosus (chronic inflammation resulting in arthritis), scleroderma (autoimmune disease resulting in hardening of the skin), polymyositis (muscle inflammation), and rheumatic fever (resulting in heart valve damage).

coronary: encircling, as the blood vessels that supply blood directly to the heart muscle; loosely used to refer to the heart and to coronary artery disease.

coronary thrombosis: presence of blood clot obstructing the flow of blood to the heart.

cortisol: a hormone of the outer layer of the adrenal gland, also called hydrocortisone.

creatinine: compound found in the blood, urine and muscle tissue. Elevated creatinine in the blood usually indicates the presence of kidney disease.

Crohn's disease: chronic inflammatory condition involving the colon and the terminal portion of the small intestines. Symptoms include abdominal pain, cramping, diarrhea, and sometimes fever and bloody stools. Complications include obstruction of the bowel, intestinal fistula, abscesses in the abdomen and around the rectum or anus, and bowel perforation (a hole in the wall of the intestine).

depression: (in psychology) dejected state of mind accompanied by feelings of hopelessness, sadness, discouragement, often with inability to function or participate in activities. The depressed person can have dramatic weight changes and sleep disturbances.

diabetes: either of two disorders—diabetes insipidus or diabetes mellitus. Insipidus denotes a metabolic disorder of the hormone system caused by a deficiency of antidiuretic hormone (ADH) normally secreted by the pituitary gland. Usually a temporary condition. Characterized by passage of large amounts of diluted, colorless urine (up to 15 quarts a day), unquenchable thirst, dry skin, and constipation. Diabetes mellitus is a chronic metabolic disorder due to insufficient insulin; symptoms include excessive thirst and urination, weight loss, excess sugar in urine and blood. Two forms of diabetes mellitus are type 1, or juvenile-onset diabetes, and type 2 or adult-onset diabetes. Treatment depends upon ability to produce insulin. *Insulin dependent:* those with an inability to produce enough insulin to process carbohydrates, fat, and protein efficiently will require insulin injections. *Non-insulin dependent:* most prevalent among obese adults. Often controlled with weight loss, exercise, and diet.

diabetic coma: result of not taking insulin properly or from the presence of stress from surgery, infection, or improper diet. Warning signs include increased thirst, vomiting, nausea, headache.

diabetic ketoacidosis: serious complication of diabetes mellitus in which the body produces acids that cause fluid and electrolyte disorders, dehydration, and sometimes coma.

diabetic retinopathy: vision disorder seen most frequently in people who have had poorly controlled insulin-dependent diabetes mellitus for several years; can lead to loss of vision.

dialysis: medical procedure for filtering waste products from the blood of some patients with kidney disease.

digitalis: a drug used to increase the force of the heart's contraction and to regulate specific irregularities of heart rhythm.

dilated cardiomyopathy: heart muscle disease that leads to enlargement of the heart's chambers, robbing the heart of its pumping ability.

diuretic: a drug that helps eliminate excess body fluid; usually used in the treatment of high blood pressure and heart failure.

Doppler studies: named after Johann Christian Doppler, Austrian scientist (1803–53) Doppler studies are measurements of systolic blood pressure using sound waves. Doppler studies are also used to measure fetal heart rate in expectant mothers.

dyspnea: shortness of breath.

echocardiogram: the record of a procedure (echocardiography) using ultrasound waves to visualize internal heart structure.

echocardiography (EEG or EKG): a test that bounces sound waves off the heart to produce pictures of its internal structures.

edema: abnormal accumulation of fluid in body tissues (swelling), in the lungs, or elsewhere.

effusion cardiac: fluid in the sac (pericardium) around the heart.

electrocardiogram (EKG or ECG): measurement of electrical activity during heartbeats.

embolism: sudden blockage of a blood vessel by an embolus (blood clot).

endocarditis: serious bacterial infection of the membrane lining of the heart and valves or heart muscle. Symptoms include fever and heart arrhythmia and can result in valve damage where surgery may be required. Those with mitral valve prolapse may be more susceptible to this condition and may have to be premedicated with antibiotic prior to dental work or surgical procedure.

endocrine disorders: any disorder involving the endocrine system. The endocrine system is made up of organs that secrete hormones into the blood to regulate basic functions of cells and tissues. Endocrine organs are pituitary, thyroid, parathyroid, adrenal glands, pancreas, ovaries (in women), and testicles (in men).

enema: introduction of a solution into the rectum and colon to stimulate bowel activity and empty the lower intestine for either feeding or therapeutic purposes, to give anesthesia, or to aid in x-ray studies.

enteroscopy: a visual examination of the inside of the intestine using a device called an enteroscope.

enzyme: a chemical originating in a cell that can act outside the cell and regulate reactions in the body.

erythropoiesis: formation of red blood cells.

erythropoietic porphyrias: inherited disorder in which there is an abnormal increase in the production of porphyrins (chemicals in all living things). Erythropoietic porphyria is characterized by production of large quantities of porphyrins in the blood-forming tissue of bone marrow. Symptoms include sensitivity to light, abdominal pain, and neuropathy.

erythropoietin (EPO): a hormone produced in the kidneys that stimulates the production of red blood cells in the bone marrow.

esophageal varices: enlarged veins on the lining of the esophagus subject to severe bleeding; often they appear in patients with severe liver disease. Symptoms include severe pain. Esophagitis inflammation of the mucous-membrane lining of the esophagus. May be caused by infection, irritation, or most commonly, from the back-flow of stomach acid.

esophagus: hollow tube that provides passage from the back of the throat to the stomach.

estrogen: the female sex hormone.

ethanol: a form of alcohol.

fasting: going without food for a period of time such as twelve-hour fasting prior to blood work.

Fe: symbol for the element iron.

fecal: pertaining to body waste, matter discharged from the bowel.

ferritin: a complex protein formed in the intestine, containing about 23 percent iron. The amount found in serum is directly related to iron storage in the body. Increased ferritin levels may indicate iron loading and conditions such as hemochromatosis, certain types of anemia, etc.

fertility: capability to reproduce.

fetal: pertaining to the fetus.

fibrocystic breast disease: presence of benign cysts in the breasts, common condition that should be monitored; reduced consumption of caffeine is recommended.

fibroids: abnormal growth of cells in the muscular wall of the uterus; uterine fibroids are composed of abnormal muscle cells and are almost always benign. Cause is unknown. Usually decreases in size without treatment after menopause.

fibromas: nonmalignant (benign) tumor of the connective tissue.

fibrosis: abnormal formation of connective or scar tissue.

fluids: non-solid, liquid or gaseous substances; secretions.

folate: folic acid.

folic acid: part of the B-complex of vitamins and needed for normal function of red and white blood cells.

FT3 (triiodothyronine): another component of thyroid hormone.

FT4 (free thyroxine): one component (1-5%) of thyroid hormone; the metabolically active part of the thyroid hormone and the more accurate indicator of thyroid function.

fungi: organisms dependent on other organisms for nourishment; a yeast, mold, or mushroom.

fulminating infection: infection that occurs suddenly and with great intensity.

gallbladder disease: any disease involving the gallbladder or biliary tract. The gallbladder is a reservoir for bile; the biliary tract is the passageway that transports bile to the small intestine. Gallbladder disease is a common, often painful condition requiring surgery. It is commonly associated with gallstones and inflammation.

gallstones: calculus or stones formed in the gallbladder.

gastrin: hormone that stimulates the production of gastric acid or stomach acid.

gastrinoma: benign or malignant gastrin-secreting islet-cell tumor of the pancreas. There is an overproduction of gastric acid often resulting in an ulcer.

gastritis: irritation, inflammation, or infection of the stomach lining. Cause is sometimes unknown but may be due to excess stomach acid, food allergy, viral infection, or adverse reaction to alcohol, caffeine, or some drug. Symptoms may include nausea, diarrhea, abdominal pain, cramps, fever, weakness, belching, bloating, and loss of appetite. Usually curable in one week if cause is eliminated.

gastroenteritis: inflammation of the stomach and intestines accompanying many digestive-tract disorders. Causes may include bacterial, viral or parasitic infections, food poisoning, food allergy, excess alcohol consumption, or emotional upset. Symptoms are the same as gastritis. Recovery usually occurs within one week. *See* gastritis.

gastrointestinal disease: any disorder of the gastrointestinal tract, which includes the mouth, esophagus, stomach, duodenum, small intestine, cecum, appendix, the ascending colon, transverse colon, descending colon, sigmoid colon, rectum, and anus.

gastrointestinal disorders: any condition or disease relating to any part of the digestive system, including the mouth, esophagus, stomach, small intestine, large intestine, and rectum. May also include some conditions relating to the liver, gallbladder, and pancreas.

gastrointestinal (GI) symptoms: any symptoms relating to the stomach or intestine. Some common GI symptoms include vomiting, diarrhea, constipation, bloating, and heartburn.

GGT (gamma glutamyl transpeptidase): an enzyme found mainly in the liver but also in many other parts of the body. Increased GGT levels are involved in hepatitis, cirrhosis, jaundice, and other disabilities.

globulins: class of proteins that are insoluble in water but soluble in saline solutions.

glucose: simple sugar that is the body's major source of energy.

glucose tolerance test: determines the body's ability to metabolize carbohydrates.

glucose-6-phosphate dehydrogenase (G6PD): an enzyme, G6PD deficiency is an inherited X-linked autosomal recessive disorder that can result in hemolytic anemia when an individual consumes fava beans or alcoholic beverages or is given certain drugs such as antimalarial or sulfa drugs. The constant hemolysis (destruction of red blood cells) leads to hemosiderosis/iron overload.

glycogen: substance formed from glucose, stored chiefly in the liver. When the blood sugar level is too low, glycogen is converted back to glucose for the body to use as energy.

gonadotropin: hormone that stimulates function of the gonads.

gonads: parts of the reproductive system that produce and release eggs (ovaries in the female) or sperm (testes in the male).

granulomas: nodule of firm tissue formed as a reaction to chronic inflammation, such as from foreign bodies or bacteria.

growth hormone (GH): a hormone regulating cell division and protein synthesis needed for normal growth.

HAA (Hepatitis-associated antigen): a protein used to detect hepatitis A and/or B virus.

HAM'S Test: an acid serum test for paroxysmal nocturnal hemoglobinuria (PNH).

haptoglobin: a protein produced by the liver. Increased haptoglobin may indicate biliary obstruction.

Hashimoto's thyroiditis: one of several kinds of thyroid gland inflammation.

HbA$_{1c}$: a monitor of the rise and fall of blood sugar over a period of time. If the blood glucose level has been carefully controlled and regulated over a period of 5-6 weeks, the HbA$_{1c}$ level will be normal; if it is elevated, it is an indication that the blood glucose level has not been controlled and has also been elevated.

HBV: hepatitis B virus, commonly known as serum hepatitis.

HCV: hepatitis C virus. Contracted from infected blood as a result of transfusion prior to July 1991, or using contaminated personal items such as razors, nail clippers, toothbrushes, syringes, tattoo needles, etc.

HDL (high-density lipoprotein): a lipoprotein produced mainly in the liver but also in the intestine; carries cholesterol to the sites where it is needed. Also called "good cholesterol."

heart attack: *See* myocardial infarction.

heart failure: loss of pumping ability by the heart, often accompanied by fatigue, breathlessness, and excess fluid accumulation in body tissues.

Heinz bodies: granular deposits in red blood cells from precipitation of proteins. They are present in certain hemolytic anemias. See anemia, hemolytic.

helicobacter pylori: a bacterium found in the cells of the stomach lining that can be a risk factor for some gastric diseases.

hematocrit (Hct): the percentage of total blood volume consisting of red blood cells, found by centrifuging the whole blood and measuring the volume of red cells in a given volume of blood. Decreased hematocrit levels are associated with anemia, hyperthyroidrism, cirrhosis, bone marrow failure, and numerous other pathogenic conditions.

hematuria: abnormal presence of blood in the urine. May be gross (can actually see the blood) or microscopic (seen only under a microscope). Is usually a sign of kidney disease or urinary tract disorder.

heme: the iron-containing portion of the hemoglobin molecule.

heme synthesis: a process where iron accumulates in the mitochondria waiting to be inserted into the heme ring of a red blood cell. The enzymatic process of heme production is complicated but essential before iron can be inserted into the heme ring to form hemoglobin. If any of these enzymes are abnormal iron accumulates resulting in iron overload condition.

hemochromatosis: genetic metabolic disorder in which excessive iron may accumulate in the liver, pancreas, heart, brain, and skin, resulting in liver disease, diabetes mellitus, heart attack, depression, impotence, and a bronze or ashen gray-green skin color.

hemoglobin (Hgb, Hb or Hbg): the iron-containing pigment of red blood cells that carries oxygen from the lungs to the tissues.

hemoglobin electrophoresis: a test that identifies blood diseases such as sickle cell disease, hemoglobin C and H disease, and thalassemia, both major and minor forms.

hemolysis: process by which red blood cells break down and hemoglobin is released. Occurs normally at the end of the life span of a red blood cell. It may also occur abnormally with certain diseases or conditions such as hemolytic anemia.

hemolytic disorder: characterized by the premature destruction of red blood cells. May or may not result in anemia, depending on the ability of the bone marrow to increase production of red blood cells.

hemolytic episode: separation of hemoglobin from red blood cells.

hemolytic jaundice: jaundice caused by severe hemolytic anemia, which results in high levels of unconjugated bilirubin. Leads to a jaundiced appearance.

hemorrhage: a severe internal or external bleeding.

hemosiderin: an iron-containing compound that is not contained in ferritin. Hemosiderin collects in vital organs such as the heart, joints, liver, lungs, brain, and pancreas, impairing function.

hemosiderosis: a condition marked by excessive iron in the tissues, especially in the liver and spleen.

heparin: an anticoagulant used in the prevention and treatment of blood clots and in the management of heart attacks.

hepatic coma: stupor or coma caused by build up of waste products in the blood that are toxic to the brain. Normally, waste products are neutralized by the liver, but due to extensive liver damage they continue to circulate in the blood.

hepatic disease: any disease involving the liver, including many types of hepatitis and cirrhosis.

hepatic dysfunction: poor liver function.

hepatitis: inflammatory liver condition.

hepatitis, acute viral: characterized by rapid onset of symptoms, loss of appetite, vomiting, fever, joint pain, and itchy skin with some forms of hepatitis; jaundice, flu-like symptoms, enlarged liver, loss of appetite, upper right quadrant abdominal pain, abnormal liver function, dark urine and clay-colored stool. Acute hepatitis can occur in all forms of viral hepatitis infection but are most common in B and C.

hepatitis A: form of viral hepatitis caused by the hepatitis. A virus that is contracted through contaminated food or water usually because of unsanitary conditions (improper hand washing after restroom use) or contaminated shellfish. A is usually mild, although it can be severe; the acute stage being about two weeks in duration. There is a hepatitis A vaccination.

hepatitis B: form of viral hepatitis caused by the hepatitis B virus that can enter the body through blood transfusions contaminated with the virus or by the use of contaminated needles or instruments. Infection may be very severe and result in prolonged illness, cirrhosis, or death. *See* cirrhosis. There is a hepatitis B vaccination.

hepatitis C: form of viral hepatitis caused by the hepatitis C virus spread through blood or sexual contact; there is no vaccine.

hepatitis, chronic: inflammation of the liver lasting more than six months; can be due to hepatitis B or C, alcohol, drugs, medications, toxic chemicals, or autoimmune conditions.

hepatocellular injury: injury of liver cells.

hepatomas: malignant tumor that begins in the liver (primary site of cancer), as opposed to liver cancer that has spread from another site.

hepatotoxicity: destructive effect on the liver usually caused by a medication or alcohol

hereditary: inherited, transmitted genetically from generation to generation.

histology: science dealing with the microscopic identification of cells and tissue.

HIV (human immunodeficiency virus): a retrovirus attacks helper T cells of the immune system and causes acquired immunodeficiency syndrome (AIDS); transmitted through sexual intercourse or contact with infected blood.

HLA (human lymphocyte antigen): existing on the surface of white blood cells, this antigen is determined genetically and is therefore useful in paternity investigation and compatibility with tissue transplantation. HLA is also useful assisting in diagnosis of other diseases, such as hemochromatosis, Reiter's syndrome, Yersinia, Graves' disease, chronic active hepatitis, juvenile diabetes, and others.

hormone: a chemical produced by a gland or tissue that is released into the bloodstream; controls body functions such as growth and sexual development. Insulin is a pancreatic hormone.

hypertension (high blood pressure): increase in the force of blood against the arteries as blood circulates through them. Often has no symptoms. Essential or primary hypertension, the most common kind, has no single identifiable cause. Secondary hypertension is caused by an underlying disease.

human growth hormone (HGH): hormone needed for normal growth and sexual maturity from birth until the end of puberty: secreted by cells in the pituitary gland.

hyper-: a prefix meaning excessive, above, or beyond.

hyperglycemia: too much sugar in the blood, as in diabetes.

hyperinsulinemia: an excessive amount of insulin in the blood.

hyperthyroidism: Over-activity of the thyroid, an endocrine gland that regulates all body functions.

hypertrophic cardiomyopathy: heart muscle disease that leads to thickening of the heart walls, interfering with the heart's ability to fill with and pump blood.

hypo-: a prefix meaning deficient, beneath, under.

hypoglycemia: a condition of low blood sugar.

hypogonadism: deficient secretion of the gonads.

hypopituitarism: a condition resulting from diminished secretion of pituitary hormone; see human growth hormone.

hypothyroidism: underactive thyroid gland, which results in decreased metabolic rate. Early symptoms may include intolerance for cold, fatigue, unexplained weight gain, constipation, and forgetfulness. The condition is caused by dysfunction of the thyroid gland and may be due to damage to the anterior pituitary, surgical removal of the thyroid, radioactive iodine treatment, Hashimoto's thyroiditis or inflammatory conditions, such as sarcoidosis. See Hashimoto's thyroiditis; sarcoidosis.

hypothyroidism, secondary: caused outside the thyroid. It may result from decreased activity of the pituitary gland, which secretes thyroid stimulating hormone (TSH), dysfunction of the hypothalamus, which regulates TSH production, iodine deficiency in the diet, or use of drugs that depress thyroid function.

hypoxia: an oxygen deficiency.

hysterectomy: surgical removal of the uterus.

idiopathic: results from an unknown cause.

IG: or immunoglobulins, IgG, IgA, IgM are tests that measure immune status.

IgG: increases in infections of all types, liver disease, myeloma and rheumatoid arthritis

IgA: increases in chronic nonalcoholic disease, primary biliary cirrhosis

IgM: increases in malaria, infectious mononucleosis, rheumatoid arthritis

ileostomy: a surgical procedure in which the lower part of the small intestine (the ileum) is cut and brought to an opening in the abdominal wall, where feces can be passed out of the body.

infarction: an infarct or area of tissue that undergoes necrosis (cell death) as a result of loss of blood supply due to an occlusion (blockage) or stenosis (narrowing or constriction).

infectious mononucleosis: infectious viral disease that affects the liver, respiratory system, and lymphatic system.

infection: the presence and growth of a microorganism that produces tissue damage.

infertility: the inability or diminished ability to produce offspring.

inflammation/inflammatory: a nonspecific immune response that occurs in reaction to any type of bodily injury. Common symptoms are pain, redness, swelling, and warmth to the injured area. Fever commonly occurs with extensive inflammation as well.

inflammatory bowel disease: a group of disorders that cause the intestines to become inflamed (red and swollen). These disorders usually last a long time and reoccur frequently. Symptoms include abdominal cramps and pain, diarrhea, weight loss, and bleeding from the intestines. Crohn's disease is one type of inflammatory bowel disease.

insulin: a hormone secreted by the beta cells of the islets of Langerhans of the pancreas that regulates blood glucose levels.

interstitial: occupies space between tissues, such as interstitial fluid.

interstitial fibrosis: formation of fibrous tissue between normal tissues.

intravenously (IV): administered through a vein.

intravenous (IV): within or into a vein.

intrinsic factor: belonging to the essential nature of a thing. SYN: inherent; innate.

iron: a metallic element widely distributed in nature. As a part of hemoglobin, iron is essential for the transport of oxygen in the blood and is also part of some of the enzymes needed for cell respiration.

iron-deficiency anemia: condition in which iron requirements exceed iron supply.

iron panel: series of tests that measure levels of iron and iron actively in the body such as amount of circulating, stored, or bound to proteins and in transport such as serum iron, transferrin, total iron binding capacity (TIBC), transferrin-iron saturation percentage, serum transferrin receptor, unbound or unsaturated iron-binding-capacity (UIBC), hemoglobin and hematocrit.

iron overload: too much iron in body, excess accumulates in vital organs resulting in disease.

ischemia: decreased blood supply to a body organ or part.

IV: intravenous.

jaundice: condition of yellow skin, yellow whites of the eyes, dark urine and light-colored stools. It is a symptom of diseases of the liver and blood caused by abnormally elevated amounts of bilirubin in the blood.

joint aspiration: the drawing off of excess fluid from around a joint by the means of suction.

juvenile: 1. Pertaining to youth or childhood. 2. Immature. In some diseases juvenile means onset prior to age thirty such as in juvenile hemochromatosis.

ketoacidosis: serious disorder that results from a deficiency or inadequate use of carbohydrates. Characterized by fluid and electrolyte disorders, dehydration, and mental confusion. If left untreated, coma and death may occur. It is usually a complication of diabetes mellitus but may also be seen in starvation and rarely in pregnancy if diet is inadequate. *See* diabetes mellitus: insulin and non-insulin dependent.

Kupffer cell: named for Karl W. von Kupffer, German anatomist. A Kupffer cell is a stellate reticuloendothelial cell that makes up the central cellular portion of the enamel organ of the dental lamina of an embryo. It is considered to give nutrition and protection to the developing enamel crown of a developing tooth.

lactoferrin: an enzyme that combines with iron in the blood causing the iron to become unavailable to many invading pathogens that require iron for their reproduction.

lamina: a thin flat layer or membrane.

LDL: low-density lipoprotein; see cholesterol.

left ventricular assist device (LVAD): a mechanical device used to increase the heart's pumping ability.

Legionnaires' disease: a severe, often fatal disease due to inhalation of certain bacillus. The disease is characterized by pneumonia, dry cough, myalgia, and sometimes gastrointestinal symptoms.

leukemia, myeloblastic: malignancy of blood cells in which the predominant cells are myeloblasts (a form of white blood cell).

libido: sexual drive or urge.

lipase: a fat-splitting enzyme found in the blood, pancreatic secretion, and tissues.

liver biopsy: procedure where a tiny sample of the liver is removed so that it can be viewed under a microscope. This procedure helps determine what is occurring in the liver and the extent of liver damage.

liver function tests: include alanine aminotransferase (ALT), also known as serum glutamic pyruvic transminase (SGPT); aspartate aminotransferase (AST), also known as serum glutamic-oxaloacetic transaminase (SGOT); gamma-glutamine transferase (GGT), alkaline phosphatase (ALP).

lung: organs of respiration. The primary purpose of the lung is to bring air and blood together so that oxygen can to added to the blood and carbon dioxide removed from it. The lungs are composed of lobes; the right lung has three and left lung has two. Lobes are divided into lobules that contain blood vessels, lymphatic nerves, and ducts that connect the alveolir air space where oxygen–carbon dioxide exchange takes place. It is in this space that alveolar macrophages can become loaded with iron when iron is inhaled.

macro-: combining form meaning large or long.

macrocytosis: a condition where cells are abnormally large.

macrophage: a monocyte (a type of white blood cell) that has left the blood stream and settled in a tissue. Macrophages are found in large quantities in the spleen, lymph nodes, alveoli, and tonsils and are one of the major cells of the immune system. About 50 percent of all macrophages are found in the liver as Kupffer cells.

malabsorption: inadequate absorption of nutrients from the intestinal tract, especially the small intestine.

malaise: vague feeling of bodily discomfort, generally prior to onset of illness.

malignant: capable of causing destruction of normal tissue; may lead to death. Usually refers to cancer growth.

maple-syrup urine disease: hereditary defect of metabolism. Usually diagnosed in infancy because it is recognized by the characteristic maple-syrup odor of urine. Other symptoms may include mental and physical retardation and feeding difficulties. *See* phenylketonuria (PKU).

MDS: myelodysplastic syndromes.

mean corpuscular hemoglobin (MCH): is the measure of the amount or weight of hemoglobin within a red blood cell; MCH part of complete blood count and helps determine types of anemia.

mean corpuscular hemoglobin concentration (MCHC): is the measure of the average concentration or percentage of hemoglobin with a single red blood cell; MCHC is part of a complete blood count and helps determine types of anemia.

mean corpuscular volume (MCV): is the measure of the average volume or size of a single red blood cell; MCV is used to determine types of anemia, liver disease, B vitamin deficiencies, alcoholism, and thalassemia.

megaloblast: a large abnormal red blood corpuscle found in the blood in cases of certain anemias.

melanoma: any of a group of malignant tumors, primarily of the skin, which develop from a pigmented mole over a period of several months or years.

metabolism: combined chemical and physical processes that take place in the body. Involves distribution of nutrients, growth, energy production, elimination of wastes, and other bodily functions. There are two phases of metabolism: anabolism, the constructive phase formation of tissues and organs; and catabolism, the breaking-down phase during which molecules are broken down.

metastasis: process by which cancerous cells or infectious germs spread from their original location to other parts of the body.

MI: myocardial infarction (heart attack).

micro-: combining form denoting small size or extent.

microbes: microorganism (small, living organism) capable of producing disease.

microcytosis: blood disorder characterized by abnormally small erythrocytes (red blood cells) often associated with iron deficiency anemia.

mitochondria: self-replicating portion of the cell where metabolic and respiratory functions provide a cell's energy source.

mitral regurgitation: defective closure of the heart's mitral valve, which allows some of the blood to back-flow or regurgitate. Normally, the mitral valve allows blood to flow from the top left chamber of the heart (atrium) to the bottom left chamber of the heart (ventricle), but prevents blood from flowing back into the left atrium. Although there are several causes, rheumatic heart disease is the single most common cause of this condition. Symptoms include fatigue and slight breathlessness. Eventually the condition may progress and result in severe congestion of the lungs. Surgery to replace or repair the mitral valve is required in patients with severe symptoms.

mitral valve: valves located in the heart between the left atrium and left ventricle.

mitral valve prolapse: condition in which the mitral valve becomes floppy, resulting in mitral regurgitation. *See* mitral regurgitation.

multiple myeloma (primary bone marrow cancer): malignancy beginning in the plasma cells of the bone marrow. Plasma cells normally produce antibodies to help destroy germs and protect against infection. With myeloma, this function becomes impaired, and the body cannot deal effectively with infection.

myocardial infarction (MI) heart attack: death of an area of heart muscle due to interruption of its blood supply. Arteries narrowed by atherosclerosis may be occluded (blocked) by blood clot (coronary thrombus). Symptoms include crushing, vise-like chest pain that may radiate especially to the left arm, neck, or jaw, shortness of breath, faintness, anxiety, ashen color, perspiration, and arrhythmia.

myoglobin: iron containing pigment that provides the red color in muscles; it also contains oxygen needed by the muscles for proper function.

myelodysplastic syndromes: a group of neoplastic diseases of the bone marrow.

neoplasm/neoplastic: a new and abnormal formation of tissue, as a tumor or growth. It serves no useful function, but grows at the expense of the healthy organism.

nephrosis: conditions in which there are degenerative changes in the kidneys or kidney disease.

neurological: Concerning the nervous system.

non-specific liver disease: poor liver function in the absence of a known cause.

normo-: combining form meaning normal or usual.

nuclear medicine scanning test: any test involving the use of radioactive substances to diagnose a number of certain conditions. The substances are either injected into the body or inhaled, the dose of radiation is minimal, and the substances used either lose their radioactivity in a short time or are excreted.

osteoporosis: a general term describing any disease process that results in reduction in bone mass.

ovaries: glands in the female that produce the reproductive cell called the ovum, and two known hormones.

ovulation: the periodic ripening and discharge of the ovum from the ovary. Ovulation occurs approximately fourteen days before the next menstrual period.

packed cells: red blood cells that have been separated from the plasma and used for conditions that require red blood cells but not the liquid components of whole blood.

pancreatitis: inflammation of the pancreas. Chronic pancreatitis usually follows recurrent attacks of acute pancreatitis. Pancreas gradually becomes unable to supply digestive juices and hormones necessary for good health.

paternal: pertaining to, or inherited from the father.

pediatric: concerning the treatment of children, i.e., those younger than age 18.

percutaneous: refers to the skin; medication by application of an ointment or removal or injection of a fluid by a needle.

pericardal: pertaining to the tissue surrounding the heart.

pernicious anemia: chronic anemia that occurs as a result of B_{12} deficiency due to the lack of intrinsic factor, a substance secreted by the mucous membranes of the stomach that is essential for absorption of B_{12}.

phlebotomy: therapeutic withdrawal of blood.

phosphates: form of inorganic phosphorus found in the body.

physicians:
- *anesthesiologist:* physician specializing in administering an anesthetic agent, usually for surgical procedures.

- *cardiologist:* physician specializing in care of disorders of the heart.

- *emergency care physician:* those treating conditions requiring immediate care.

- *endocrinologist:* physician specializing in care and treatment of all types of disorders of the ductless glands.

- *family practitioner:* a physician whose care is for the entire range of diseases affecting persons of all ages and sexes and not limited to a particular organ system or disease; a general practitioner.

- *gastroenterologist:* a physician whose practice covers disorders of the stomach, intestines, and related structures such as the esophagus, liver, gallbladder, and pancreas.

- *general practitioner:* see family practitioner.

- *hematologist:* a physician specializing in the study of blood and in the diagnosis and treatment of disorders of the blood and blood-forming tissues.

- *hepatologist:* a specialist in diseases of the liver.

- *internist:* a physician specializing in internal medicine.

- *nephrologist:* a physician concerned with the structure and function of the kidneys.

- *neurologist:* a specialist in diseases of the nervous system.

- *rheumatologist:* a specialist in rheumatic diseases of the joints.

- *pediatrician:* a physician treating children and children's diseases.

- *psychiatrist:* a physician who specializes in the study, treatment, and prevention of mental disorders.

- *psychologist:* a specialist, studying and treating disorders of the mental processes that affect behavior.

- *pulmonary physician:* a physician whose practice is concerned or involved with the lungs.

phytates: compounds found in whole grains that prevent over-absorption of iron.

plasma: the liquid part of the blood and of the lymph.

platelets: a round or oval disk found in the blood.

polycythemia: increase in red blood cells in the body. The disease has three forms. Polycythemia vera involves overproduction of red blood cells, white blood cells, and platelets. Secondary polycythemia is a complication of diseases or factors other than blood cell disorders. Stress polycythemia involves decreased blood plasma.

polycythemia vera: overproduction of red blood cells, white blood cells, and platelets. Cause is unknown. Treatment may include withdrawing blood at certain intervals, radioisotope therapy, and drug therapy. Treatment is needed to prevent blood clots from forming that could cause a stroke, heart attack, or blockage in a vein or artery.

porphyria: excretion of porphyrins into the urine.

porphyria, acute intermittent (AIP): rare inherited disorder characterized by excessive formation and excretion of porphyrins. See porphyrins. Symptoms include recurrent abdominal pain often accompanied by nausea, vomiting, constipation, and dark urine.

porphyria cutanea tarda: inherited metabolic disorder involving the synthesis of red pigment (heme) in blood cells due to a defective enzyme (uroporphyrinogen decarboxylase) in the liver, which results in an increase in porphyrins in the skin. Increased porphryins lead to photosensitivity where the skin is damaged by sunlight. This type of porphyria usually associated with chronic alcoholism marked by skin lesions and enlarged liver. *See* porphyria, acute intermittent.

porphyrins: any number of pigments widely distributed in living tissue; found in hemoglobin and myoglobin.

portal shunt: transjugular intrahepatic portosystemic shunt (TIPS). A flexible stent composed of an expandable stainless-steel mesh that is inserted through the jugular vein and fed down through the portal vein. The shunt is used to help maintain pressure in the portal vein in those with esophageal varices, a life-threatening condition of bleeding varices.

protein: one of a class or kind of complex compound synthesized by all living things, which provides the amino acids essential for growth and repair of tissue.

protein metabolism: process by which protein foods are used by the body to make tissue proteins, together with breaking down tissue proteins to produce energy. Food proteins are first broken down into amino acids then absorbed into the blood and finally used in body cells to form new proteins. Diseases affecting protein metabolism include liver disease, maple-sugar urine disease (due to the color of urine), and phenylketonuria (PKU).

pruritus: itching.

PSA (prostate-specific antigen): an antigen found in all males, greatly increased in cases of prostate cancer.

pulmonary: concerning or involving the lungs.

pulmonary congestion (or edema): fluid accumulation in the lungs.

quantitative phlebotomy: removal of a certain amount of blood as advised by the physician.

radiography: the process of obtaining an x-ray.

RBC: red blood cells.

RDW (red blood cell distribution width): an indication of the variation in red blood cell size.

red cell indices: blood test that provides important information about the size, hemoglobin concentration, and hemoglobin weight of an average blood cell. Aids in classification of anemias. Indices include mean corpuscular volume (MCV), mean corpuscular hemoglobin (MCH), and mean corpuscular hemoglobin concentration (MCHC). MCV expresses the average size of many cells and indicates whether most red blood cells are undersized (microcytic), oversized (macrocytic), or normal sized (normocytic). MCH is the hemoglobin-to-red-blood-cell ratio and gives the weight (concentration) of hemoglobin in an average red blood cell. MCHC defines the volume of hemoglobin in an average red cell and helps distinguish normally colored (normochromic) red blood cells from pale (hypochromic) red cells.

reductase: an enzyme that accelerates the reduction process of chemical compounds.

renal: pertaining to the kidneys.

restrictive cardiomyopathy: heart muscle disease in which the muscle walls become stiff and lose their flexibility; typically results from another disease elsewhere in the body such as amyloidosis (abnormal protein fibers accumulate in the heart muscle), sarcoidosis (inflammatory diseases that causes the formation of small lumps in organs) and hemochromatosis/iron overload.

reticulocytes: young, immature red blood cells.

reticulocytosis: excess amount of reticulocytes in the blood.

reticuloendothelial system (RES): body system involved primarily in defense against infection and in disposal of products of the breakdown of cells. Made up of cells that are able to surround, engulf, and digest microorganisms and cell debris (macrophages) and special cells in the liver, lungs, bone marrow, spleen, and lymph nodes.

rheumatic fever: inflammatory disease occurring primarily in children as a result of delayed reaction to streptococcal throat; may result in rheumatic heart disease, heart muscle and valve damage.

rheumatoid arthritis: inflammatory condition characterized by joint disease that involves muscles, cartilage, and membrane linings of the joints. Three times more common in women than men. Symptoms include red, warm, painful joints usually symmetric, i.e., affects both sides. Sometimes accompanied by weakness and fatigue. If disease is severe, permanent deformity and crippling may result.

sarcoidosis: chronic inflammatory disease of unknown origin that causes the formation of small lumps (nodules) in organs.

septum: partition or dividing wall in an organ; in the heart, a muscle wall separating chambers.

sero-negative rheumatoid arthritis: test for rheumatoid factor is negative, common in iron-related arthritis.

serum: the watery portion of the blood left after clotting is completed.

SGOT (serum glutamic-oxaloacetic transaminase): a test used in cases of suspected coronary occlusive heart diseases or liver diseases such as hepatitis or cirrhosis.

SGPT (serum glutamic-pyruvic transaminase): an enzyme released into the bloodstream by injury or disease affecting the liver.

sickle cell anemia, disease trait: a condition in which each red blood cell contains both normal and abnormal hemoglobin.

sideroblastic anemia: a disorder in which incorporation of iron into hemoglobin and the developing red blood cells (erythroblasts) in the bone marrow is faulty. As a result, iron accumulates in the erythroblasts giving rise to ringed sideroblasts, which when found on microscopic examination of bone marrow provide diagnosis. Because ring sideroblasts develop poorly or not at all into mature red cells, anemia is the consequence (the red blood cells of the mitochondria are overloaded with iron) and hemoglobin production (heme synthesis) is defective. Acts like iron deficiency anemia (IDA), but unlike IDA in that iron testing is normal or increased.

sideroblasts: young red blood cells that contain excess iron.

Sjogren's syndrome : an autoimmune disorder characterized by dryness of the eyes and mouth and recurrent salivary gland enlargement.

sleep apnea: the stopping of breathing during sleep for a duration of at least ten seconds.

sperm count: the measure of the number of sperm in a precise volume of fluid.

steatohepatitis: fatty liver.

stool occult blood: a measure of the presence of more than minimal amounts of blood in a stool sample; may indicate abnormalities in the gastrointestinal tract.

sudden death: cardiac arrest caused by an irregular heartbeat.

sudden infant death: death of unknown cause in infants under six months of age.

sugar levels: *see* blood sugar; glucose.

synovial: pertaining to the synovia, the lubricating fluid of the joints.

synovial syndrome: abnormal value or finding within the synovial (joint) fluid.

synovium: synovial membrane.

T3e: triiodothyronine, one of two forms of thyroid hormone.

T4: thyroxine, one of the principal hormones secreted by the thyroid gland.

tachycardia: heartbeat that is too fast.

testosterone: the principal male hormone, produced in the testes.

thalassemia: name for a complex of hereditary anemias that occur in populations bordering the Mediterranean and in Southeast Asia.

therapeutic: a healing agent or results obtained from treatment.

thyroid gland: large endocrine gland located in the throat area, which produces a hormone that regulates metabolism.

thyroid profile: blood tests performed to determine thyroid function, include T3 uptake and T4 uptake, Free thyroxine Index (T7), Thyroid stimulating hormone (TSH), Thyrotropin.

thyroiditis: inflammation of the thyroid gland. Acute thyroiditis is caused by a bacterial infection and often results in formation of abscesses. Subacute thyroiditis usually follows a viral infection and is characterized by sore throat, fever, weakness, and a painful, enlarged thyroid gland.

tomography: an x-ray technique that selects a particular level in the body and blurs out structures above and below that plane. It gives a clear image of the selected plane of the body.

total iron binding capacity (TIBC): a measurement of all proteins available for binding free iron in the body; an indirect but accurate measure of transferrin (see transferrin). Increased TIBC levels may indicate iron-deficiency anemia; a decreased TIBC may indicate cirrhosis or several types of anemia.

transferrin: protein that transports iron from the intestine into the blood. It makes iron available to the bone marrow, where red blood cells are produced.

TRH (thyrotropin-releasing factor): substance secreted by the hypothalamus that controls the release of thyroid-stimulating hormone (TSH) from the anterior pituitary gland.

triglycerides (TGs): a form of fat in the blood stream, produced in the liver.

TSH (thyroid-stimulating hormone): substance secreted by the anterior pituitary gland that controls the release of thyroid hormone from the thyroid gland. TSH is needed for normal thyroid growth and function. *See* thyroid gland.

tumor: a spontaneous new growth of tissue that forms an abnormal mass and does not follow normal laws of growth; may be malignant or nonmalignant.

tumor marker: a substance in blood serum whose presence may indicate a possible malignancy.

ulcer: an open sore on the skin or on a mucous membrane that may have a variety of causes such as stress, bacteria, a specific disease, etc.

ultrasound: the use of very high-frequency sound waves to produce an image or photograph of an organ or tissue.

unbound or unsaturated iron-binding capacity (UIBC): there are three components to the iron binding capacity of serum:
- Serum iron is the concentration of iron present. Normal range is 40–180 mcg/dL.
- Total iron binding capacity (TIBC) is the maximum amount of iron that can be bound. Normal range is 250–450 mcg/dL.
- The unsaturated iron binding capacity (UIBC) is the difference between the TIBC and the serum iron. Normal range is 70–390 mcg/dL. Iron-binding capacity levels TIBC and UIBC are high in anemias and low in iron overload.

upper gastrointestinal (UGI): a means of obtaining a direct look at the upper gastrointestinal tract by using a long, flexible fiberoptical scope.

urea: a substance formed in the liver and found in blood, lymph, and urine; the end product of protein metabolism in the body.

vascular: pertaining to blood vessels.

ventricles: the two lower chambers of the heart. The left ventricle is the main pumping chamber in the heart.

ventricular fibrillation: rapid, irregular quivering of the heart's ventricles, with no effective heartbeat.

vibrio: a member of a genus of gram-negative bacilli that can be found in raw shellfish or contaminated water; these can be deadly to someone with high iron levels.

viral: caused by a virus.

WBC: white blood cells.

Wilson's disease: inherited disorder of copper metabolism in which copper accumulates in the liver, red blood cells, and brain, which leads to anemia, tremors, liver dysfunction, and dementia.

x-ray: a name for a machine using the energy of electromagnetic waves to visualize hard tissues such as bone, or a treatment with such a machine.

Yersinia: a gram negative bacteria.

zinc: a metallic element and an essential element in the diet of all animals, including humans. Lack of zinc in the diet can cause slowing of growth or healing of wounds among other things, and during pregnancy may cause developmental disorders in the child.

Contacts

We have endeavored to include organizations that might be helpful to a person with hemochromatosis and consequential disease. Any organization missing from this list may contact us at comments@irondisorders.org to notify us of changes and updates for contact information.

Alopecia (Balding)
National Alopecia Areata Foundation
710 C Street, Suite 11
San Rafael, CA 94901
415-456-4644
e-mail: naaf@compuserve.com

Alcoholism
Al-anon Family Group Headquarters
1600 Corporate Landing Parkway
Virginia Beach, VA 23454
800-356-9996; 757-563-1600
http://www.al-anon.alateen.org

Alcoholics Anonymous
P.O. BOX 459, Grand Central Station
New York, NY 10163
212-870-3400
http://www.alcoholics-anonymous.org

National Clearinghouse for Alcohol and Drug Information
P.O. Box 2345
Rockville, MD 20847
800-729-6686; 301-468-2600
http://www.health.org

National Council on Alcoholism and Drug Dependence
12 West 21st Street
New York, NY 10010
800-NCA-CALL; 212-206-6770
http://www.ncadd.org

Arthritis
American Juvenile Arthritis Organization
1314 Spring Street NW
Atlanta, GA 30309
800-283-7800; 404-872-7100

Ankylosing Spondylitis Association
P.O. Box 5872
Sherman Oaks, CA 91413
800-777-8189
http://www.spondylitis.org

Arthritis Foundation
1330 W. Peachtree Street
Atlanta, GA 30309
800-283-7800; 404-872-7100
http://www.arthritis.org

Blood Disorders
Aplastic Anemia & MDS International
800-747-2820

Leukemia Society of America
600 Third Street
New York, NY 10016
800-955-4LSA; 212-573-8484
http://www.leukemia.org

MDS Foundation
800-637-0839

National Association for Sickle Cell Disease
2000 Corporate Point, Suite 495
Culver City, CA
800-421-8453; 310-216-6363

National Cooley's Anemia Foundation
(16 Chapters)
129-09 26th Avenue
Flushing, NY 11354
800-522-7222; 718-321-2873
www.thalassemia.org

Stroke and Neurological Disorders
National Institute of Neurological Disorders and Stroke
Office of Science and Health Reports
P.O. BOX 5801
Bethesda, MD 20824
800-352-9424; 301-496-5751
http://www.ninds.nih.gov

Alzheimer's Association
919 Michigan Ave.
Suite 1000
Chicago, IL 60611-1676
800-272-3900; 312-335-8700
http://www.alz.org

Cancer
American Cancer Society
1599 Clifton Road NE
Atlanta, GA 30329-4251
800-ACS-2345; 404-320-3333
http://www.cancer.org

National Cancer Institute
Cancer Information Service
9000 Rockville Pike
Bethesda, MD 20892
800-4-CANCER; 301-496-5583

Cardiovascular Disorders
American Heart Association
7272 Greenville Avenue
Dallas, TX 75231
214-373-6300
http://www.americanheart.org

National Heart, Lung, and Blood Institute
Information Center
P.O. Box 30105
Bethesda, MD 20824-0105
301-251-1222

National Stroke Association
96 Inverness Drive East, Suite 1
Engelwood, CA 80112
800-787-6537; 303-649-9299
e-mail: info@stroke.org
http://www.stroke.org

Deafness and Hearing Disorders
American Tinnitus Association
P.O. Box 5
Portland, OR 97207
503-248-9985
e-mail: tinnitus@ata.org

National Association of the Deaf
814 Thayer Avenue
Silver Spring, MD 20910
301-587-1788; 301-587-1789
http://www.nad.org

Death and Bereavement
Hospice Education Institute
190 Westbrook Road
Essex, CT 06426
800-331-1620; 860-767-1620
e-mail: hospiceall@aol.com

National Hospice Organization
1901 N. Moore Street, Suite 901
Arlington, VA 22209
800-658-8898; 703-243-5900
e-mail: drsnho@cais.com
http://www.nho.org

Diabetes
American Diabetes Association
1600 Duke Street
Alexandria, VA 22314
800-232-3472; 703-549-1500
http://www.diabetes.org

Juvenile Diabetes Foundation International
120 Wall Street, 19th Floor
New York, NY 10005
800-223-1138
http://www.jdfcure.com

National Diabetes Information Clearinghouse
One Information Highway
Bethesda, MD 20892-3560
301-654-3327
http://www.niddk.nih.gov

Prevent Blindness America
500 East Remington Road
Schaumburg, IL 60173
800-331-2020; 312-843-2020
e-mail: 74777.100@compuserve.com
http://www.prevent-blindness.org

The American Amputee Foundation, Inc.
Executive Assistant
P.O. Box 250218
Hillcrest Station
Little Rock, AR 72225
501-666-2523

Digestive Disorders
Crohn's and Colitis Foundation of America
386 Park Avenue South, 17th Floor
New York, NY 10016
800-343-3637
http://www.ccfa.org

Digestive Disease National Coalition
507 Capitol Court NE, Suite 200
Washington, DC 20002
202-544-7497

International Foundation for Gastrointestinal Function Disorder
P.O. Box 17864
Milwaukee, WI 53217
869-964-2001; 414-964-1799
http://www.execpc.com/iffgd

Intestinal Disease Foundation
1323 Forbes Avenue, Suite 200
Pittsburg, PA 15219
412-261-5888

National Digestive Diseases Information Clearinghouse
Two Information Highway
Bethesda, MD 20892-3570
301-654-3810

Disabilities and Rehabilitation
Disabled American Veterans
National Headquarters
3725 Alexanderia Park

Cold Springs, KY 41076
606-441-7300
http://www.dav.org

National Organization on Disability
2100 Pennsylvania Avenue NW
Washington, DC 20037
202-293-5960
http://www.nod.org

National Rehabilitation Information Center
8455 Colesville Road, Suite 935
Silver Springs, MD 20910
800-346-2742
http://www.naric.com/naric

Endocrine Disorders
Thyroid Foundation of America
Ruth Sleeper Hall; Room RSL350
40 Parkman Street
Boston, MA 02114
617-726-8500
http://www.mssm.edu/medicine/endocrinology

Pituitary Tumor Network Association
16350 Ventura Blvd. #231
Encino, CA 91436
800-642-9211; 805-499-9973
e-mail: ptna@pituitary.com
http://www.pituitary.com

Epilepsy
Epilepsy Foundation of America
4351 Garden City Drive
Landover, MD 20785
800-450-EFA; 301-459-3700
e-mail: postmaster@efa.org
http://www.efa.org

General

The American Medical Association
515 North State Street
Chicago, IL 60610
312-464-5000
http://www.ama-assn.org

The Center for Disease Control and Prevention
1600 Clifton Road NE
Atlanta, GA 30333
404-639-3311
http://www.cdc.gov

National Institutes of Health
9000 Rockville Pike
Bethesda, MD 20892
301-496-4000
http://www.nih.gov

Restless Legs Syndrome Foundation
819 Second Street SW
Rochester, Minnesota 55902-2985
website: www.rls.org
e-mail: mailtoRLSFoundation@rls.org
507-287-6465

U.S. Department of Health and Human Services
200 Independence Avenue SW
Washington, DC 20201
202-619-0257
http://www.os.dhhs.gov

U.S. Food and Drug Administration
Office of Consumer Affairs Inquiry
Information Line
301-827-4420
http://www.fda.gov

Genetic Conditions
The Alliance for Genetic Support Groups
800-336-GENE (4363) or
http://www.geneticalliance.org

Greenwood Genetics Center
1 Gregor Mendel Circle
Greenwood, SC 29646
864-941-8100
888-GGC-GENE; 888-442-4363

National Society of Genetic Counselors at
610-872-7608
http://www.nsgc.org

University of Mississippi Medical Center
2500 North State Street
Jackson, MS 39215
Christopher A. Friedrich, M.D., Ph.D.
Associate Professor, Dept. of Preventive Medicine
Clinic phone number: 601-984-1900

University of Pennsylvania Hemochromatosis Clinic
Medical Genetics Division
Department of Medicine
Hospital of the University of Pennsylvania
1 Maloney Bldg.
Philadelphia, PA 19104-4283
215-662-4740
http://www.med.upenn.edu/penngen/

Hemochromatosis/Iron Overload
International Contacts
We wish to thank Philip deSterke for an excellent list of international links; visit the Dutch/Netherlands website
http://members.tripod.com/~hemochromatose/
p_de_sterke@hotmail.com

Australia
Haemochromatosis Society Australia Inc.
412 Musgrave Road Coopers Plains
Phone: 07 3345 7583 Fax: 07 3345 8051
P.O. Box 154, Coopers Plains 4108
e-mail: haemsoc@gil.com.au
www.gil.com.au/~haemsoc/index.html

Canada
The Canadian Hemochromatosis Society
272-7000 Minoru Blvd.
Richmond, BC
Canada V6Y 3Z5
1-877-BAD-IRON (1-877-223-4766) Toll-Free In Canada only.
604-279-7135: Fax: 604-279-7138
e-mail: chcts@istar.ca

France
French Hemochromatosis Association
e-mail: hemochromatose@wanadoo.fr

Great Britain
The UK Haemochromatosis Society
Hollybush House, Hadley Green, Barnet, Herts, ENS 5P, England
Tel: 0181 449 1363 Email ghsoc@compuserve.com

Ireland
Irish Haemochromatosis Society
1 Upper Cherryfield avenue
Ranelagh, Dublin 6
tel: 087-232 91 09
e-mail: irhaem@hotmail.com

United States
American Hemochromatosis Society
1-888-655-IRON (4766)
www.americanhs.org

Community Blood Center of the Ozarks
2230 S. Glenstone Ave.
Springfield, MO 65804
417-227-5000

HemoCenter Rochester NY
University of Rochester Medical Center
601 Elmwood Avenue
Rochester, NY 14642
716-275-2100
http://www.urmc.rochester.edu

Hemochromatosis Foundation, Inc.
P.O. Box 8569
Albany, NY 12208
518-489-0972

Iron Disorders Institute
P.O. Box 2031
Greenville, SC 29602
864-292-1175
www.irondisorders.org
irondis@aol.com
comments@irondisorders.org

Iron Overload Diseases Association
433 Westwind Drive
North Palm Beach, FL 33408-5123
407-840-8512

Kaiser Permanente, San Diego California
Hospital and Medical Offices
4647 Zion Ave.
San Diego, CA 92120
619-528-5000
http://www.kaiserpermanente.org

Mayo Clinic
200 First Street SW
Rochester, MN 55905
507-284-2511
http://www.mayo.edu

Oklahoma Blood Institute
1001 N. Lincoln Boulevard
Oklahoma City, OK 73104
405-297-5700
http://www.obi.org

Reading Hospital System
Sixth Avenue and Spruce Street
P.O. Box 16052
Reading, PA 19612-6052
610-988-8201
http://www.readinghospital.org

Red Cross National Testing Laboratory - Atlanta
1890-F Beaver Ridge Circle
Norcross, GA 30071
770-798-8000

University of Alabama
UAB Hospital
619 19th Street South
Birmingham, AL 35249
http://www.health.uab.edu

University of Massachusetts Memorial Medical Center
Memorial Campus
281 Lincoln Street
Worcester, MA 01605
508-793-6611
http://www.umassmed.edu

University of Pennsylvania Treatment Center
Department of Medicine

Division of Medical Genetics
3400 Spruce Street
Philadelphia, PA 19104
215-662-4740

University of Washington, Seattle
Iron Disorders Clinic, Dr. Kris Kowdley
1959 NE Pacific St.
Seattle, WA 89195-6174
206-598-4886

Impotence
Impotents Anonymous
119 South Ruth Street
Maryville, TN 37803-5746
615-983-6092

Infertility
Ferre Institute, Inc.
258 Genesee Street, Suite 302
Utica, NY 13502
315-724-4348

Kidney Disorders
American Association of Kidney Patients
100 S Ashley Drive, Suite 280
Tampa, FL 33602
800-749-2257
e-mail: aakpnat@aol.com
http://www.aakp.org

National Kidney Foundation
30 East 33rd Street, Suite 1100
New York, NY 10016
800-622-9010; 212-889-2210
http://www.kidney.org

National Kidney and Urologic Diseases
Information Clearinghouse
Three Information Way
Bethesda, MD 20892-3580
301-654-4415
http://www.niddk.nih.gov

Learning Disabilities
National Center for Learning Disabilities
381 Park Avenue South, Suite 1420
New York, NY 10016
212-545-7510

Liver Disorders
American Liver Foundation
1425 Pompton Avenue
Cedar Grove, NJ 07009
800-223-0179; 201-256-2550

Hepatitis Foundation International
American Porphyria Foundation
P.O. Box 22712
Houston, TX 77227
713-266-9617

Medic Alert
Medic Alert Foundation International
P.O. Box 1009
Turlock, CA 95381
800-432-5378

Pain Relief
American Chronic Pain Association
P.O. Box 850
Rocklin, CA 95677
916-632-0922

National Chronic Pain Outreach Association
7979 Old Georgetown Road, Suite 100
Bethesda, MD 20814
301-652-4948

Travel Health
Information Travelers Hotline Centers for Disease Control
and Prevention
404-332-4559

Bibliography

Adams, P. "Prevalence of Abnormal Iron Studies in Heterozygotes for Hereditary Hemochromatosis." *American Journal of Hematology* 45 (1994): 146–49.

———. "Alcohol in Hereditary Hemochromatosis Additive Hepatoxic Effect." *Hepatology* 23 (1996): 724.

———. "Factors Affecting the Rate of Iron Mobilization During Venesection Therapy for Genetic Hemochromatosis." *American Journal of Hematology* 58 (1998):16–19.

———. Population Screening for Haemochromatosis. *Gut* 46 (2000): 301–3.

Andrews, N. C., and J. E. Levy. "Iron is Hot: An Update on the Pathophysiology of Hemochromatosis." *Blood* 92 (1998): 1845–51.

Anthone, S., C. Ambrus, R. Kohli, I. Min, R. Anthone, A. Stadler, I. Stadler, and A. Vladutiu. "Treatment of Aluminum Overload Using a Cartridge with Immobilized Desferrioxamine." *Journal of the American Society of Nephrology* 6 (1995): 1271–77.

Aust, A., L. Lund, C. Chao, S. Park, and R. Fang. "Role of Iron in the Cellular Effects of Asbestos." *Inhalation Toxicology* 12 (2000): 75S–80S.

Barton, J. C., E. H. Barton, L. F. Bertoli, C. H. Gothard, and J. S. Sherrer. "Intravenous Iron Dextran Therapy in Patients with Iron Deficiency Anemia and Normal Renal Function Who Failed to Respond to or Did Not Tolerate Oral Iron Supplementation." *The American Journal of Medicine*, 109 (2000): 27–32.

Beard, J. L., "Iron Requirements in Adolescent Females." *Journal of Nutrition* 130 (2000): 440S–442S.

Beutler, E. "Targeted Disruption of the HFE Gene." *Proceedings of The National Academy of Sciences, USA* 95 (1998): 2033–34.

———, V. Felitt, T. Gelbart, and N. Ho. "The Effect of HFE Genotypes on Measurements of Iron Overload in Patients Attending a Health Appraisal Clinic." *Annals of Internal Medicine* 133 (2000): 329–37.

Bonkovsky, H. L., and J. V. Obando. "Role of HFE Gene Mutations in Liver Diseases Other than Hereditary Hemochromatosis." *Current Gastroenterology Reports* 1 (1999): 30–37.

———, R. B. Rubin, E. E. Cable, A. Davidoff, T. H. Pels Rijcken, and D. D. Stark. "Hepatic Iron Concentration: Noninvasive Estimation by Means of MR Imaging Techniques." *Radiology* 21 (1999): 227–34.

Bothwell, T. H., and A. P. MacPhail. "Hereditary Hemochromatosis: Etiologic, Pathologic, and Clinical Aspects." *Seminars in Hematology* 35 (1998): 55–71.

Burke, W., E. Thomson. M. Khoury, S. McDonnell, N. Press, P. Adams, J. Barton, E. Beutler, G. Brittenham, A. Buchanan, E. Clayton–Wright, M. Cogswell, E. Meslin, A. Motulsky, L. Powell, E. Sigal, B. Wilfond, and F. Collins. "Hereditary Hemochromatosis: Gene Discovery and Its Implications for Population Based Screening." *JAMA* 280 (1998): 172–78.

Brandhagen, D. J., V. F. Fairbanks, W. P. Baldus, C. I. Smith, K. E. Kruckeberg, D. J. Schaid, and S. N. Thibodeau. "Prevalence and Clinical Significance of HFE Gene Mutations in Patients with Iron Overload." *American Journal of Gastroenterology* 95 (2000): 2910–14.

Brittenham, G. M., A. L. Franks, and F. R. Rickles. "Research Priorities in Hereditary Hemochromatosis." *Annals of Internal Medicine* 129 (1998): 993–96.

Camaschella, C., A. Roetto, M. Cicilano, P. Pasquero, S. Bosio, L. Gubetta, F. Di Vito, D. Girelli, A. Totaro, M. Carella, A. Grifa, and P. Gasparini. "Juvenile and Adult Hemochromatosis are Distinct Genetic Disorders." *European Journal of Human Genetics* 5 (1997): 371–75.

———, A. Roetto, A. Cali, M. De Gobbi, G. Garozzo, M. Carella, N. Majorano, A. Totaro, and P. Gasparini. "The Gene TFR2 is Mutated in a New Type of Haemochromatosis Mapping to 7q22." *Nature Genetics* 25 (2000): 14–15.

Centers for Disease Control and Prevention. "Recommendations to Prevent and Control Iron Deficiency in the United States." *MMWR* 47 (1998): 1–28.

Conlon B. J., and D. W. Smith. "Supplemental Iron Exacerbates Aminoglycoside Otoxicity In Vivo." *HearingResearch* 115 (1998): 1–5.

Cook, J. D., C. A. Finch, and N. J. Smith. "Evaluation of the Iron Status of a Population." *Blood* 48 (1976): 449–55.

———, B. S. Skikne, S. R. Lynch, and M. E. Reusser. "Estimates of Iron Sufficiency in the US Population." *Blood* 68 (1986): 726–31.

Crawford, D. H. G., E. C. Jazwinska, L. M. Cullen, and L. W. Powell. "Expression of HLA-Linked Hemochromatosis in Subjects Homozygous or Heterozygous for the C282Y Mutation." *Gastroenterology* 114 (1998): 1003–08.

Crosby, W. H. "A History of Phlebotomy Therapy for Hemochromatosis." *The American Journal of The Medical Sciences* 301 (1991): 28–30.

Dalhoj, J., H. Kiaer, P. Wiggers, R. W. Grady, R. L. Jones, and A. S. Knisely. "Iron Storage Disease in Parents and Sibs of Infants with Neonatal Hemochromatosis: 30 Year Follow-up." *American Journal of Medical Genetics* 37 (1990): 342–45.

Dreyfus, J. "Lung Carcinoma Among Siblings Who Have Inhaled Dust Containing Iron Oxides During Their Youth." *Clinical Medicine* 30 (1936): 256–60.

Failla, M, C. Giannattasio, A. Piperno, A. Vergani, A. Grappiolo, G. Gentile, E. Meles, and G. Mancia. "Radial Artery Wall Alterations in Genetic Hemochromatosis Before and After Iron Depletion Therapy." *Hepatology* 32 (2000): 569–73.

Felitti, V. J. "Hemochromatosis: A Common, Rarely Diagnosed Disease." *The Permanente Journal* 3 (1999): 10–22.

Forge, A., and J. Schacht. "Aminoclycoside Antibiotics." *Audiology Neurootology* 5 (2000): 3–22.

Franks, A. L., and W. Burke. "Will the Real Hemochromatosis Please Stand Up?" *Annals of Internal Medicine* 130 (1999): 1018–19.

Garcia, A. R., R. J. Montali, J. L. Dunn, N. L. Torres, J. A. Centeno, and Z. Goodman. "Hemochromatosis in Captive Otarids" (Proceedings AAZV and IAAAM Joint Conference, 2000), 197.

Garcia-Casal, M. N., I. Leets, and M. Layrisse. "Beta–Carotene and Inhibitors of Iron Absorption Modify Iron Uptake by Caco-2." *Cell Journal of Nutrition* 130 (2000) : 5–9.

Ghio, A. J., R. J. Pritchard, K. L. Dittrich, and J. M. Samet. "Non-heme (Fe3+) in the Lung Increases with Age in Both Humans and Rats." *Journal of Laboratory and Clinical Medicine* 129 (1997): 53–61.

Goodnough, L. T., B. Skikne, and C. Brugnara. "Erythropoietin, Iron, and Erythopoiesis." *Blood* 96 (2000): 823–833.

Guillen, C., I. B. McInnes, D. Vaughan, A. B. J. Speekenbrick, and J. H. Brock. "The Effects of Local Administration of Lactoferrin on Inflammation in Murine Autoimmune and Infectious Arthritis." *Arthritis and Rheumatism* 43 (2000): 2073–80.

Harmatz, P., E. Butensky, K. Quirolo, R. Williams, L. Ferrell, T. Moyer, D. Golden, L. Neumayr, and E. Vichinsky. "Severity of Iron Overload in Patients with Sickle Cell Disease Receiving Chronic Red Blood Cell Transfusion Therapy." *Blood* 96 (2000): 76–79.

Harris, Z. L., Y. Takahashi, H. Miyajima, M. Serizawa, R. MacGillivray, and J. Gitlin. "Aceruloplasminemia: Molecular Characterization of this Disorder of Iron Metabolism." *Proceedings National Academy of Sciences USA* 92 (1995): 2539–43.

———, A. Durley, T. Man, J. Gitlin. "Targeted Gene Disruption Reveals an Essential Role for Ceruloplasmin in Cellular Iron Efflux." *Proceedings National Academy Sciences USA* 96 (1999): 10812–17.

Kaltwasser, J. P., R. Gottschalk, and C. H. Seidl. "Severe Juvenile Hemochromatosis (JH) Missing HFE Gene Variants: Implications for a Second Gene Locus Leading to Iron Overload." *British Journal of Haematology* 102 (1998): 1111–12.

Kamp, D. W., V. A. Israbian, A. V. Yeldand, R. J. Panos, P. Graceffa, and S. A. Weitzman. "Phytic Acid, an Iron Chelator, Attenuates Pulmonary Inflammation and Fibrosis in Rats after Intratracheal Instillation of Asbestos." *Toxicologic Pathology* 23: (1995): 689–95.

———, M. J. Greenberger, J. S. Sbalchierro, S. E. Preusen, and S. A. Weitzman. "Cigarette Smoke Augments Asbestos–Induced Alveolar Epithelial Cell Injury: Role of Free Radicals." *Free Radical Biology and Medicine* 25 (1998): 728–39.

Knisely, A. S. "Neonatal Hemochromatosis." *Advances in Pediatrics* 39 (1992): 383–403.

Kiechl, S., J. Willeit, G. Egger, W. Poewe, and F. Oberhollenzer. "Body Iron Stores and the Risk of Carotid Atherosclerosis." *Circulation* 96 (1997): 3300–07.

Klipstein-Grobusch, K., J. F. Koster, D. E. Grobbee, J. Lindermans, H. Boeing, A. Hofman, and C. M. Witterman. "Serum Ferritin and Risk of Myocardial Infarction in the Elderly: The Rotterdam Study." *American Journal of Clinical Nutrition* 69 (1999): 1231–36.

Kuryshev, Y.A., G. M. Brittenham, H. Fujioka, P. Kannan, C. C. Shieh, S. A. Cohen, and A. M. Brown. "Decreased Sodium and Increased Transient Outward Potassium Currents in Iron-Loaded Cardiac Myocytes." *Circulation* 100 (1999): 675–83.

Lamarche, J. B., M. Cote, and B. Lemieux. "The Cardiomyopathy of Friedreich's Ataxia Morphological Observations in Three Cases." *Canadian Neurological Science* 7 (1980): 389–96.

Lapenna, D., S. De Gioia, A. Mezzett, G. Ciofani, A. Consoli, L. Marzio, and F. Cuccurullo. "Cigarette Smoke, Ferritin, and Lipid Peroxidation." *American Journal of Respiratory Critical Care Medicine* 151 (1995): 431–35.

Lauffer, R. *Iron and Your Heart.* (New York: St. Martin's Press, 1991).

Layrisse, M., M. Garcia-Casal, L. Solano, M. Baron, F. Arguello, D. Llovera, J. Ramierz, I. Leets, and E. Tropper. "Iron Bioavailability in Humans from Breakfasts Enriched with Iron Bis-Glycine Chelate, Phytates and Polyphenols." *Human Nutrition and Metabolism* 9 (2000): 2195–99.

Leigh, M.J., and D. D. Miller. "Effects of pH and Chelating Agents on Iron Binding by Dietary Fiber: Implications for Iron Availability." *The American Journal of Clinical Nutrition* 38 (1983): 202–13.

Lonnerdal, B. "Effects of Milk and Milk Components on Calcium, Magnesium, and Trace Element Asborption During Infancy." *Physiological Reviews* 77 (1997): 643–69.

Looker, A. C., M. Loyevsky., and V. R. Gordeuk. "Increased Serum Transferrin Saturation Is Associated with Lower Serum Transferrin Receptor Concentration." *Clinical Chemistry* 45 (1999): 2191–99.

Mateos, F., J. Brock, and J. L. Perez-Arellano. "Iron Metabolism in the Lower Respiratory Tract." *Thorax* 53 (1998): 594–600.

McCord, J. M. "Effects of Positive Iron Status at a Cellular Level." *Nutritional Reviews* 54 (1996): 85–88.

———. "Iron, Free Radicals and Oxidative Injury." *Seminars in Hematology* 35 (1998): 5–12.

McDonnell, S. M., P. D. Phatak, V. Felitti, A. Hover, and G. D. McLaren. "Screenings for Hemochromatosis in Primary Care Settings." *Annals of Internal Medicine* 129 (1998): 962–970.

McDonnell, S. M., D. L. Witte, M. E. Cogswell, and R. McIntyre. "Strategies To Increase Detection of Hemochromatosis." *Annals of Internal Medicine* 129 (1998): 987–92.

———, B. L. Preston, S. A. Jewell, J. C. Barton, C. Q. Edwards, P. Adams, R. Yip. "A Survey of 2,851 Patients with Hemochromatosis: Symptoms and Response to Treatment." *American Journal of Medicine* 106 (1999): 619–24.

Meyers, D.G., D. Strickland, P. A. Maloley, J. K. Seburg, J. E. Wilson, and B. F. McManus. "Possible Association of a Reduction in Cardiovascular Event with Blood Donation." *Heart* 78 (1997): 188–93.

Meyers, D. G., D. McCall, T. D. Sears, T. S. Olson, and G. L. Felix. "Duplex Pulsed Doppler Echocardiography in Mitral Regurgitation." *Journal of Clinical Ultrasound* 14 (1986): 117–21.

Montosi, G, P. Paglia, C. Garuti, C. A. Guzman, J. M. Bastin, M. P. Colombo, and A. Pietrangelo. "Wild-type HFE Protein Normalizes Transferrin Iron Accumulation in Macrophages from Subjects with Hereditary Hemochromatosis." *Blood* 96 (2000): 1125–29.

Morck, T. A., S. R. Lynch, and J. D. Cook. "Inhibition of Food Iron Absorption by Coffee. "*The American Journal of Clinical Nutrition* 37 (1983): 416–20.

Muller-Berghaus, J., A. S. Knisely, R. Zaum, A. Vierzig, E. Kirn, D. V. Michalk, and B. Roth. "Neonatal Haemochromatosis: Report of a Patient with Favorable Outcome." *European Journal of Pediatrics* 156 (1997): 296–98.

Niederau, C. "Iron Overload and Atherosclerosis." *Hepatology* 32 (2000): 672–74.

O'Brien, K. O., N. Zavaleta, L. E. Caulfield, J. Wen, and S. A. Abrams. "Prenatal Iron Supplements Impair Zinc Absorption in Pregnant Peruvian Women." *Journal of Nutrition* 130 (2000: 2251–55.

O'Brien-Ladner, A. R., S. R. Nelson, W. J. Murphy, B. M. Blumer, and L. J. Wesselius. "Iron Is a Regulatory Component of Human Il-1B Production." *American Journal of Respiration and Cell Molecular Biology* 23 (2000): 112–19.

Olivieri, N F. "The Thalassemias." *New England Journal of Medicine* 341 (1999): 99–109.

———, G. M. Brittenham, C. E. McLaren, D. M. Templeton, R. G. Cameron, R. A. McClelland, A. D. Burt, and K. A. Fleming. "Long-term Safety and Effectiveness of Iron-Chelation Therapy with Deferiprone for Thalassemia Major." *New England Journal of Medicine* 339 (1998): 417-23.

Pietrangelo, A. "EASL International Consensus, Conference on Haemochromatosis." *Journal of Hepatology* 33 (2000): 485–504.

Phatak, P. D., R. L. Sham, R. F. Raubertas, K. Dunnigan, M. T. O'Leary, C. Braggins, and J. D. Cappuccio. "Prevalence of Hereditary Hemochromatosis in 16,031 Primary Care Patients." *Annals of Internal Medicine* 129 (1998): 954–61.

Qian, M., and J. Eaton. "Glycochelates and the Etiology of Diabetic Peripheral Neuropathy." *Hypothesis Paper* 28 (2000): 652–56.

Roetto, A., F. Alberti, F. Daraio, A. Cali, M. Cazzola, A. Totaro, P. Gasparini, and C. Camaschella. "The Juvenile Hemochromatosis Locus Maps to Chromosome 1q." *American Journal of Human Genetics* 64 (1999): 1388–93.

Roughead, Z. K., and J. R. Hunt. "Adaptation in Iron Absorption: Iron Supplementation Reduces Nonheme-Iron but not Heme-Iron Absorption from Food." *American Journal of Clinical Nutrition* 72 (2000): 982–89.

Rosmorduc, O., R. Poupon, I. Nion, D. Wendum, J. Feder, G. Bereziat, and B. Hermelin. "Differential HFE Allele Expression in Hemochromatosis Heterozygotes." *Gastroenterology* 119 (2000): 1075–86.

Salonen, J. T, K. Nyyssonen, H. Korpela, J. Tuomilehto, R. Seppanen, and R. Salonen. "High Stored Iron Levels are Associated with Excess Risk of Myocardial Infarction in Eastern Finnish Men." *Circulation* 86 (1992): 802–811.

Schumacher, R. H., P. C. Straka, M. A. Krikker, and A. T. Dudley. "The Arthropathy of Hemochromatosis." *Annals New York*

Academy of Sciences 526 (1988): 224–33.

Sheth, S., and G. M. Brittenham. "Genetic Disorders Affecting Proteins of Iron Metabolism: Clinical Implications." *Annual Reviews Medicine* 51 (2000): 443–64.

Siimes, M. A. "Hematopoeisis and Storage of Iron in Infants." In *Iron Metabolism in Infants*, edited by B. Lonnerdal, Boca Raton: CRC Press, 1990, 34–62.

Stephansson, O., P. Dickman, A. Johansson, and S. Cnattingius. "Maternal Hemoglobin Concentration During Pregnancy and Risk of Stillbirth." *JAMA* 284 (2000): 2611–17.

Umbreit, J. N., M. E. Conrad, E. G. Moore, and L. F. Latour. "Iron Absorption and Cellular Transport: The Mobilferrin/Paraferritin Paradigm. *Seminars in Hematology* 35 (1998): 13–26.

Varkonyi, J., J. P. Kaltwasser, C. Seidl, G. Kollai, H. Andrikovics, and A. Tordai. "A Case of Non-HFE Juvenile Hemochromatosis Presenting with Adrenocortical Insufficiency." *British Journal of Haematology* 109 (2000): 248–53.

Weinberg, E. D. "Iron and Susceptibility to Infectious Disease." *Science* 184 (1974): 952–56.

———. "The Role of Iron in Cancer." *European Journal of Cancer Prevention* 5 (1996): 19–36.

———. "Iron Withholding: A Defense Against Viral Infections." *Biometals* 9 (1996): 393–99.

Wesselius, L. J., I. M. Smirnov, M. E. Nelson, A. R. O'Brien–Ladner, C. H. Flowers, and B. S. Skikne. "Alveolar Macrophages Accumulate Iron and Ferritin After In Vivo Exposure to Iron or Tungsten Dusts." *Journal Laboratory and Clinical Medicine* 127 (1996): 401–09.

Witte, D., W. Crosby, C. Edwards, V. Fairbanks, and F. Mitros. "Hereditary Hemochromatosis." *Clinica Chimica Acta* 245 (1996): 139–200.

Ye, Z., and J. Connor. "Screening of Transcriptionally Regulated Genes Following Iron Chelation in Human Astrocytoma Cells." *Biochemical and Biophysical Research Communications* 264 (1999): 709–13.

Zacharski, L. R., D. L. Ornstein, S. Woloshin, and L. M. Schwartz. "Association of Age, Sex, and Race with Body Iron Stores in Adults: Analysis of NHANES III Data." *American Heart Journal* 140 (2000): 98–104.

Index

E-F

G-H

I-K